FUTURE AGENDA
Open Foresight

FUTURE OF PATIENT DATA

Insights from Multiple Expert Discussions Around the World

Contents

Foreword	6
Acknowledgements	7
Introduction	8
Context	16
Shared Challenges	**26**
Integration	28
Ownership vs. Access	38
Trust	45
Security and Privacy	52
Future Opportunities	**60**
Personalisation	62
Data Marketplaces	70
The Impact of AI	75
New Models	88
Emerging Issues	**98**
Data Sovereignty	100
Digital Inequality	104
Privatisation of Health Information	113
The Value of Health Data	117
Conclusions	122
Questions	124
Appendix	126

Charts

Project Summary	10
Healthcare Spend vs Life Expectancy	12
Growth In Healthcare Data	17
Doctors with EHR and Multifunctional Health IT Capacity	30
Consumers Willing To Share Health Data	46
Data Breach Cost Per Capita	53
World's Biggest Data Breaches	54
Number of Personalised Medicines (US - 2008 to 2016)	65
Genetic Disorders with Diagnostic Tests Available	67
Number of Artifical-Intelligence Companies	78
Older Adults With Three Or More Chronic Conditions	106

Case studies

Validic	35
Apple	36
Nebula Genomics	43
Digi.me	44
Flatiron	50
Deepmind	82
iCarbonX	84
Facebook	86
Verily	94
Amazon	96
Cityblock	111
Tricog	112

Foreword

It is clear that we are witnessing a growing revolution around the provision of healthcare. In the main this is being driven by the proliferation of medical data and the technology that supports this. As the pressures on existing healthcare providers continue to escalate, the better collection, management and use of more patient-specific information provides a significant opportunity for innovation and change. In the winter of 2017/18 the Future Agenda team made this the focus of our latest Open Foresight project and this led us to hold 12 discussions across 11 countries and gather outlooks from over 300 experts.

During these discussions there was near universal agreement that there are significant opportunities to be explored and, within this, few are blind to the challenges ahead. Better diagnosis, the ability to manage or delay the onset of chronic conditions, driving cost reductions and enabling greater, more personalised patient focus are just some examples of the upsides. However, at the same time, concerns were raised around the difficulty of integration of multiple datasets, the need to improve trust amongst all parties, the complexities of data ownership and in ensuring the overall security of personal information.

It is also noticeable that there are several important emerging issues that are the source of major differences of opinion around the world. How to best accommodate rising data sovereignty concerns, the privatization of health information and the growing value of health data are just three examples.

Some of the challenges and opportunities are technical in nature, but many are concerned with different ethical, philosophical and cultural approaches to health and how we treat the sick in society. We suggest that these, in particular, can best be solved through the provocation of thoughtful debate and by the collaborative sharing of views across multiple regions and sectors.

As with all Future Agenda projects we have done our best to engage with many different and alternative voices in different geographies and are delighted that so many leading organisations have supported this approach. We hope that this document is an accurate reflection of what we heard and, that by sharing the observations, it generates new ideas and inspires different approaches to solve some of the future challenges and so improve healthcare.

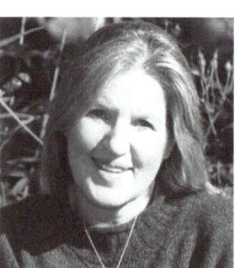

Caroline Dewing
co-Founder

caroline.dewing@futureagenda.org

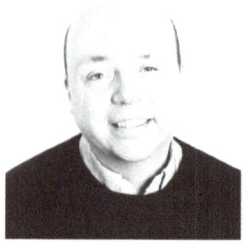

Dr Tim Jones
co-Founder

tim.jones@futureagenda.org

Acknowledgements

The insights upon which this report is based were gained via multiple discussions with over 300 experts around the world. We would also like to thank all those who have spared their time to join in these events and share their perspectives.

We hope that this report provides an accurate reflection of your views. In addition, we would like to thank the generosity of the forward-looking organisations that have supported the varied events.

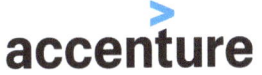
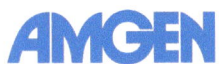
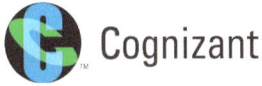
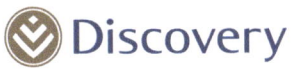
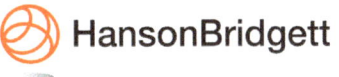
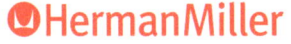
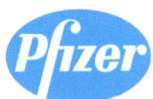
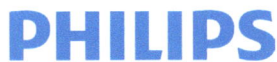
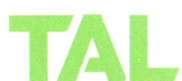
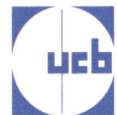
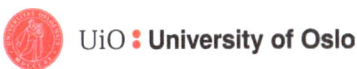
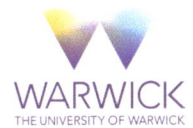
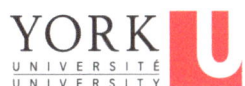

Introduction

The world's healthcare systems are experiencing significant change. We are at a point, or more accurately multiple points, of major transition around the ways we can improve access, manage and transform how to control and treat disease. The expectation is that over the next few years we will see a sizeable shift in the effectiveness of healthcare.

As the impact of rising public expectation around better wellness and health, the effect of increasingly sedentary lifestyles and progressively aging populations all converge, some fear that, in many nations, we will be unable to find the necessary funds for high quality healthcare. Others are more hopeful that with the adoption of new technologies, particularly associated with a more patient-centric approach to both health and sick care, we are on the cusp of a significant step forward in the efficiency, efficacy and effectiveness of how we diagnose, treat, manage and, ideally, prevent chronic and acute disease. Indeed, a commonly shared ambition is that a more information-rich, digital approach to healthcare over the next decade will inherently be more effective and patient focussed.

Some key advances that are seen to have already had substantial effect include:

- Wider adoption of smartphones which are able to sense as well as diagnose,
- More empowered patients equipped with a burgeoning volume of information about their condition,
- Tangible advances in machine learning, cognitive computing and wider AI,
- Increasing automation across healthcare – from chat-bots to surgery,
- The expansion of wearables, providing access to new aspects of personal health data and
- A steady decrease in the cost of, and an increase in, the access to genetic profiling.

Within this context, there are however many differences of opinion and perspectives on how these and other shifts will actually play out over the next decade. What will drive them? Who will pay? Who will benefit the most? How quickly will transformation occur? What will be the catalysts for change? Where specifically will be the greatest impact and why? These are all key questions that many organisations around the world and across multiple sectors are asking. As many governments, companies and communities all seek to make the right moves and investments, a good number are keen to see the global, cross-functional context within which the possible change is occurring. In a sector where fragmentation is sometimes extreme, where funding is often challenging and where local or regional regulations can frequently influence the market, many are keen to gain the broader perspective and then see how, where and why their individual areas of focus can have the greatest impact.

Approach

In order to provide a global view of the patient data arena, over a six-month period the Future Agenda team undertook a major multi-country project to explore the key changes on the horizon. A series of 12 events took place around the world from September 2017 to the end of January 2018 providing the opportunity to discuss the major shifts with multiple experts from across a wide range of industries, providers, researchers, governments and start-ups.

As with all Future Agenda programmes, each event brought together a rich mix of informed people who could challenge existing assumptions, share new perspectives and build insightful pragmatic views of how change will most likely occur. Starting with an initial perspective drawn from existing research and previous discussions about the future of health, the future of ageing, the future of data and the future of privacy, this series of workshops progressively identified the key issues that matter, added in additional views and highlighted the pivotal areas for future innovation and the most significant shifts - both globally and locally. Each event was supported and hosted by different organisations from across the healthcare arena keen to collaborate and build the informed global view. This report is a synthesis of the insights gained from these discussions.

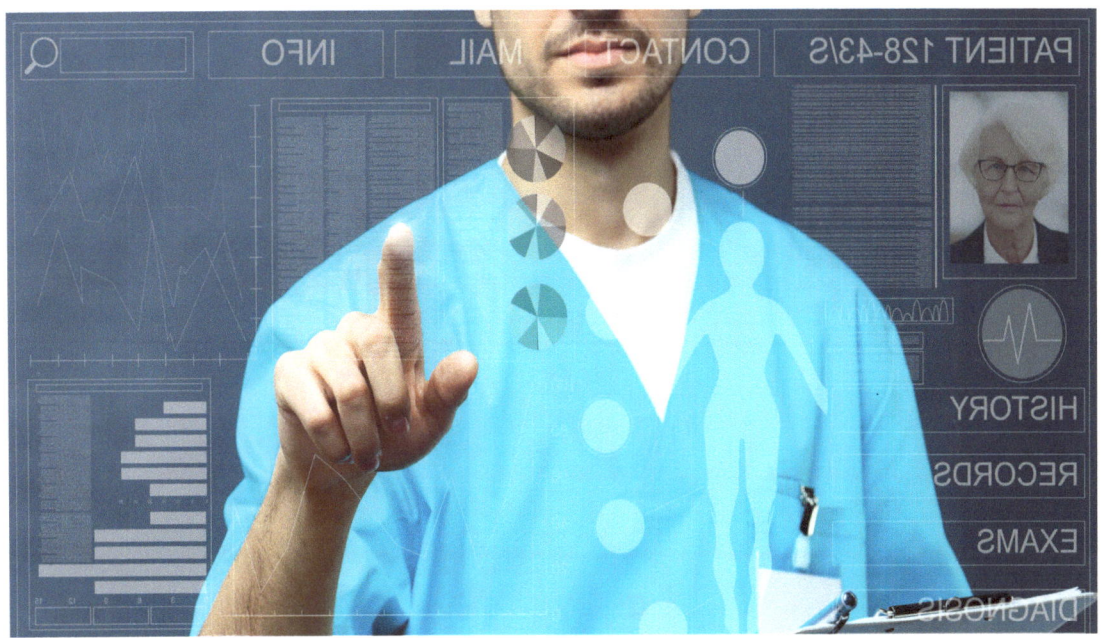

Project Summary

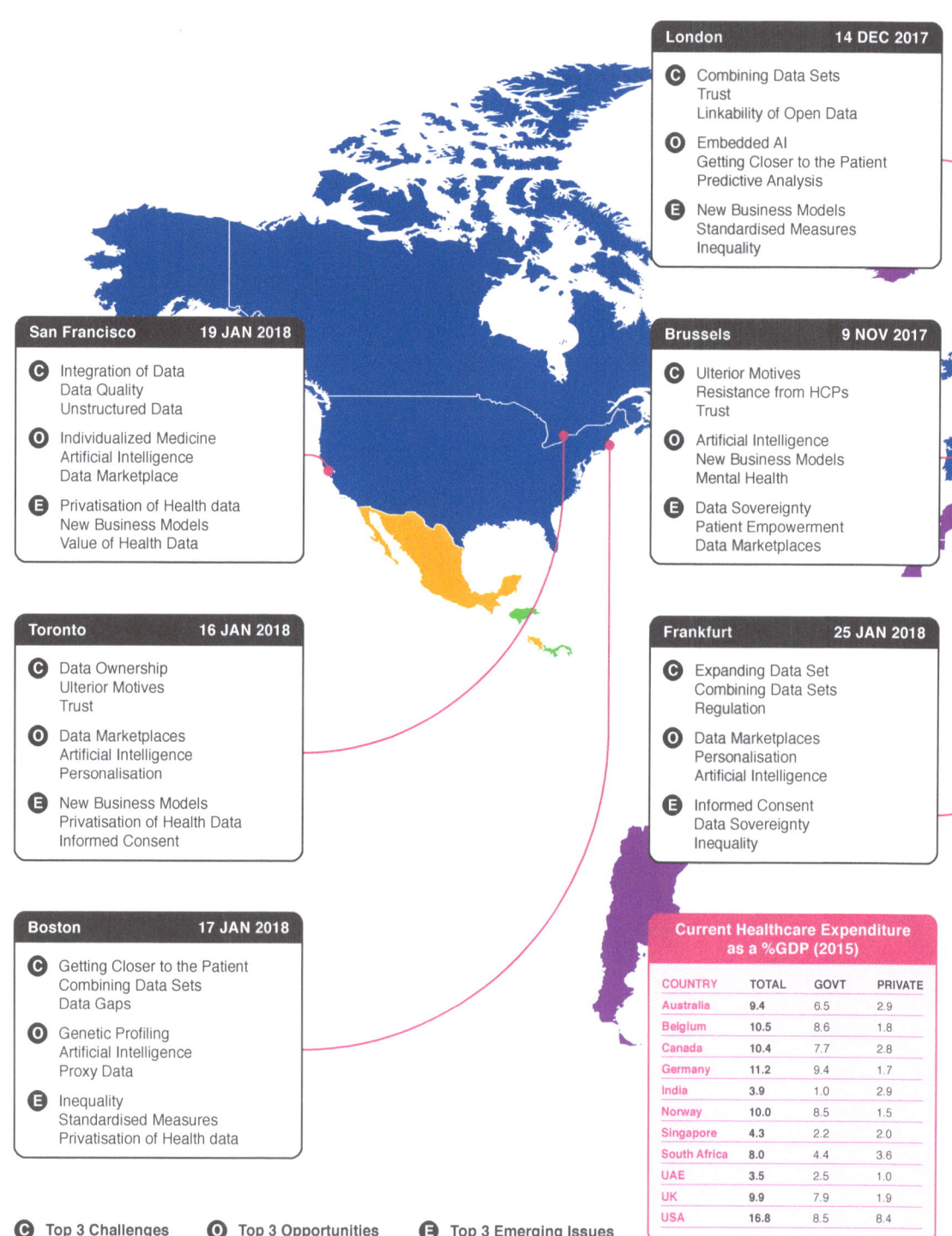

London — 14 DEC 2017
- **C** Combining Data Sets / Trust / Linkability of Open Data
- **O** Embedded AI / Getting Closer to the Patient / Predictive Analysis
- **E** New Business Models / Standardised Measures / Inequality

San Francisco — 19 JAN 2018
- **C** Integration of Data / Data Quality / Unstructured Data
- **O** Individualized Medicine / Artificial Intelligence / Data Marketplace
- **E** Privatisation of Health data / New Business Models / Value of Health Data

Brussels — 9 NOV 2017
- **C** Ulterior Motives / Resistance from HCPs / Trust
- **O** Artificial Intelligence / New Business Models / Mental Health
- **E** Data Sovereignty / Patient Empowerment / Data Marketplaces

Toronto — 16 JAN 2018
- **C** Data Ownership / Ulterior Motives / Trust
- **O** Data Marketplaces / Artificial Intelligence / Personalisation
- **E** New Business Models / Privatisation of Health Data / Informed Consent

Frankfurt — 25 JAN 2018
- **C** Expanding Data Set / Combining Data Sets / Regulation
- **O** Data Marketplaces / Personalisation / Artificial Intelligence
- **E** Informed Consent / Data Sovereignty / Inequality

Boston — 17 JAN 2018
- **C** Getting Closer to the Patient / Combining Data Sets / Data Gaps
- **O** Genetic Profiling / Artificial Intelligence / Proxy Data
- **E** Inequality / Standardised Measures / Privatisation of Health data

C Top 3 Challenges **O** Top 3 Opportunities **E** Top 3 Emerging Issues

Current Healthcare Expenditure as a %GDP (2015)

COUNTRY	TOTAL	GOVT	PRIVATE
Australia	9.4	6.5	2.9
Belgium	10.5	8.6	1.8
Canada	10.4	7.7	2.8
Germany	11.2	9.4	1.7
India	3.9	1.0	2.9
Norway	10.0	8.5	1.5
Singapore	4.3	2.2	2.0
South Africa	8.0	4.4	3.6
UAE	3.5	2.5	1.0
UK	9.9	7.9	1.9
USA	16.8	8.5	8.4

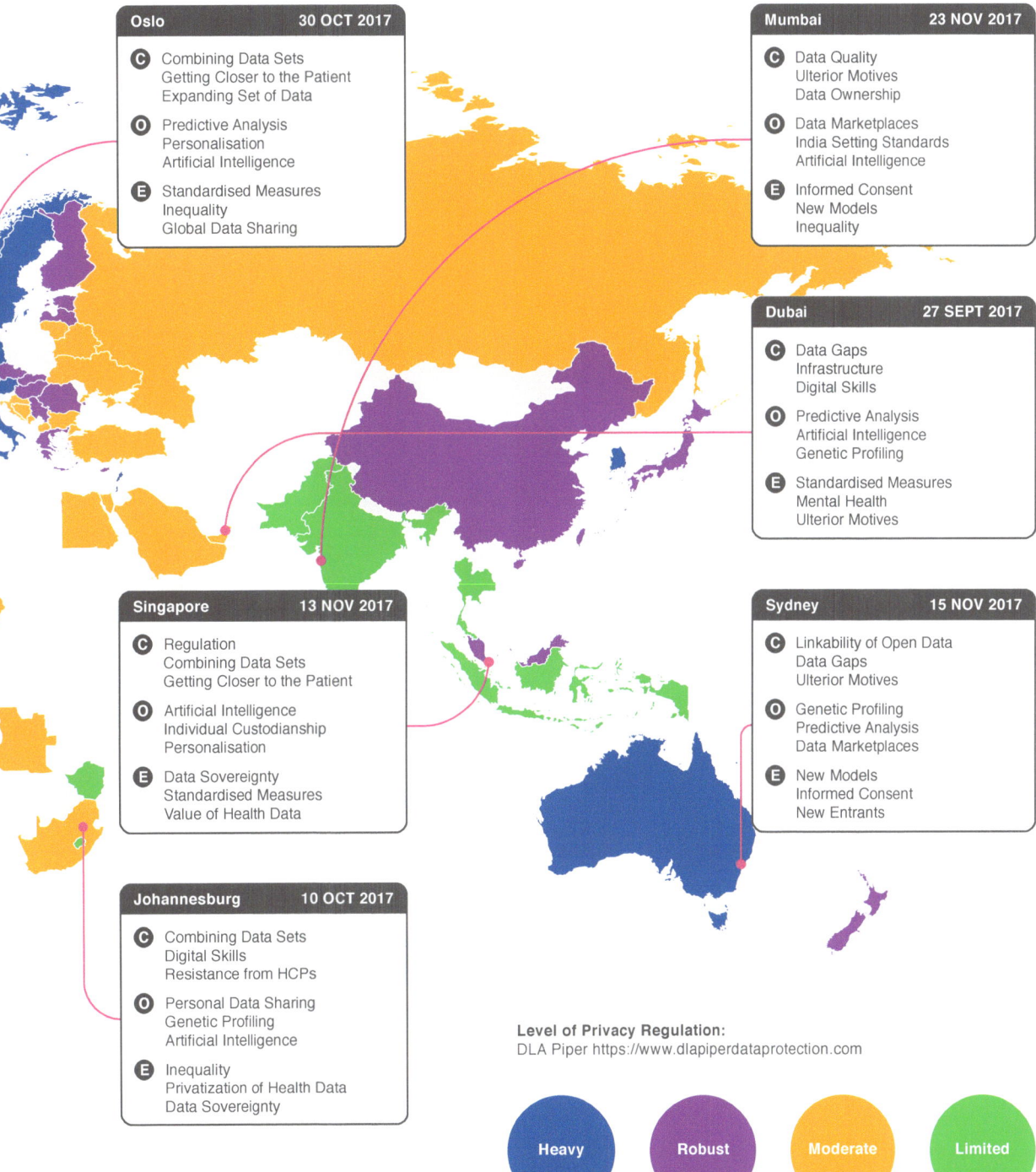

Locations and hosts

In order to gain a diverse range of perspectives we chose to hold the discussions in a variety of countries where healthcare is at different stages of evolution, where funding systems and access to funding vary and where regulation around privacy, and patient data in particular, is taking alternative paths. This is highlighted in the preceding Project Summary and in the Healthcare Spend vs Life Expectancy chart below.

Healthcare Spend vs Life Expectancy

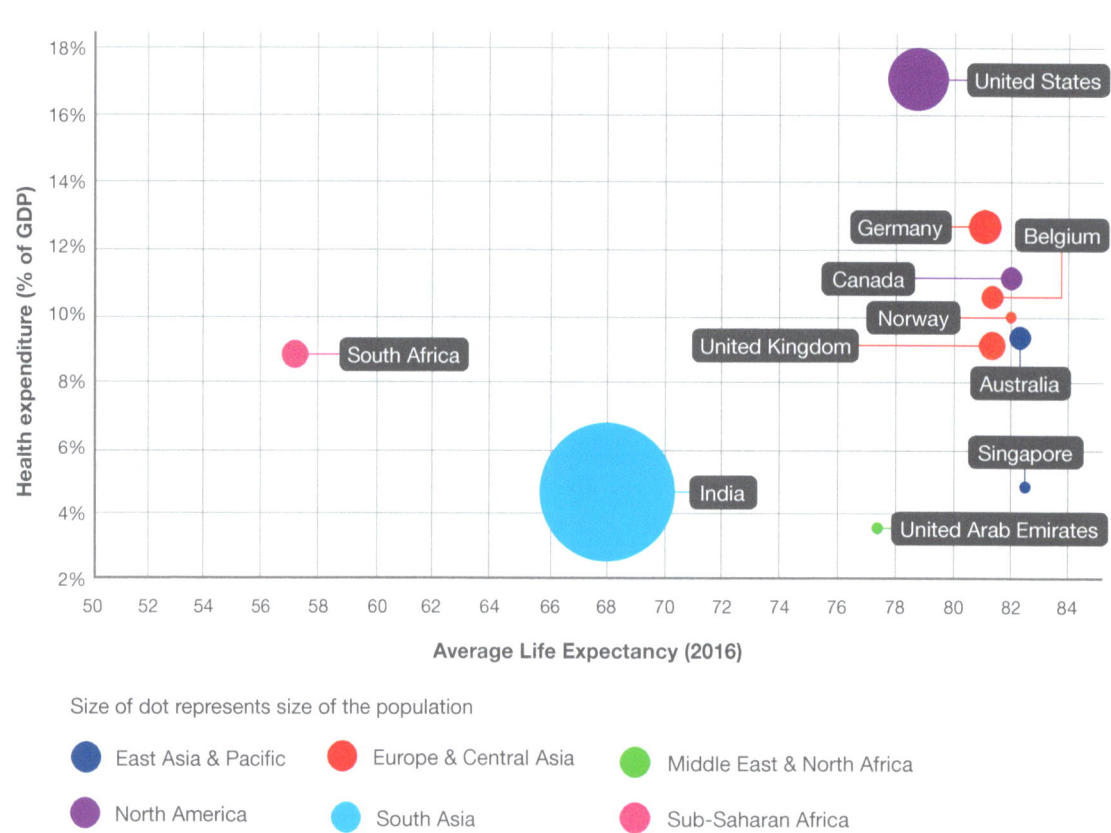

We kicked the project off in September 2017 in **Dubai** in the UAE, one of the wealthiest nations in the Middle East with a small population of 6.0 million and an average life expectancy of 77.7 years. It is also a country with high-levels of government control and significant inequality between the rich Emiratis, the wealthy ex-pats and the poorer migrant workers. It also has a relatively low overall healthcare spending of 3.5% of GDP but this figure does not include the informal care provided by domestic staff. This opening event was hosted by Herman Miller.

In early October we moved onto **Johannesburg** in South Africa, a far poorer country. It has 1/6th of the GDP per capita of the UAE and an average life expectancy of just 57 years. Its total healthcare spending of 8.0% of GDP is almost evenly split 55/45 between public and private systems but, according to the national government,[1] most of the private healthcare is focused on just 16% of the population. This event was hosted by Discovery Health.

Next, we went to **Oslo** in Norway, one of the wealthiest and, arguably, the healthiest country of all. With life expectancy of 82 years and healthcare spend running at 10% of GDP, Norwegians are also seen by many measures to be consistently among of the happiest and best educated in the world. Beyond this, Norway is in the top 5 most 'digital' nations. This workshop was the first of three supported by Accenture and took place at the University of Oslo.

In November, our focus shifted to **Brussels** to gain both the Belgian and the wider EU policy perspective. With an average life expectancy of 81 years and healthcare spend also of 10% GDP, Belgium is one of the wealthier European countries. Its GDP per capita is just over $41,000 compared to the EU which collectively has a GDP per capita of around $39,000 and average life expectancy of 80.2 years. The Brussels workshop was hosted by UCB.

Then, we moved to **Singapore**, another very wealthy, highly digital but relatively small 5.8m population nation with strong government influence over many aspects of life and the economy. With, at 83 years, the highest average life expectancy of all the countries we visited, official healthcare spend is relatively low, at 4.3%. However, as with the UAE, this does not include a significant proportion of the informal care provided by domestic staff. The event here was also hosted by Accenture.

Sydney was the next port of call. Despite the Australia's physical size, its total population is just over 24m. With an overall GDP per capita of $50,000, similar to that of Singapore, and a healthcare spend of 9.5% of GDP split 2 to 1 between public and private systems, Australia is also one of the world's healthier nations with an average life expectancy just over 82 years. The Sydney workshop was jointly hosted by TAL and Pfizer.

The last event of November was held in **Mumbai**, one of India's largest cities. With a rapidly growing population now over 1.3bn, India is moving fast up many global rankings around technology and health. Although, on average, still a poor country with the lowest GDP per capita of the nations visited and average life expectancy of 68.3 years, healthcare spend is rising and is currently at 3.9% of GDP. While these figures may give a view of a poor country, it is important to remember that India also has some of the wealthiest people in the world and so, given the size of the population and economy overall, the 2.9% of GDP spend on private healthcare is globally significant.

In December the final workshop of 2017 was in **London** where the dominant NHS single payer system is seen as one of the most efficient in the world. Although often portrayed in the media as being under stress, in a country of 70m, the UK is spending just under 10% of its GDP on a healthcare system, 80% of which is via the NHS, and is achieving average life expectancy of 81 years. This event was the third supported by Accenture and was hosted by the University of Warwick in London.

13

In January the focus moved to North America; first to **Toronto** in Canada. Another vast country with a population of only 36m, Canada is also seen to be one of the healthier global nations. Average life expectancy is just under 82 years and its healthcare spend is 10.5% GDP, of which over 70% is in the hands of the public sector. The Toronto event was hosted by York University.

Next, we moved to the US - first to **Boston** and then to **San Francisco**. With, at around 17% of GDP, the highest healthcare spending in the world, there is little doubt of the influence of the US market on global healthcare. However, with over 50% of this focused on the private system and over 12% of the total 325m population now without any insurance cover, there is also significant health inequality. The Boston workshop was supported by Amgen and hosted by Philips and the San Francisco event was hosted by Hanson Bridgett.

The final workshop of this project took place in **Frankfurt** in Germany. With one of Europe's most advanced healthcare systems, average life expectancy is currently 80.8 years and healthcare spend is over 11% of GDP with 84% of this provided from government. The home of many leading medical equipment and pharmaceutical companies, Germany also has a significant influence on the global market. This event was hosted by Cognizant.

Report structure

From these 12 discussions and additional dialogue in New York, Singapore and London, we have explored many points of view hearing different perspectives on some pivotal issues that may well have a major impact on how change will play out across healthcare in the next 10 years.

There has also been clear areas of consensus around where and why we may see the greatest shifts in the use of patient data taking place. This document provides a summary of the insights and, at its core, is based on the views of over 300 experts, entrepreneurs and other informed individuals who attended our events. It is a playback of what we heard in the varied discussions with additional research and context added to help frame some of the primary points made.

We have structured this report into 5 sections:

- **Context** – addressing the growing sources and users of patient data as well as the global ambition
- **Shared Challenges** – that are seen as common issues to address across multiple locations
- **Future Opportunities** – highlighted as priority areas in the varied discussions
- **Emerging Issues** – that will become increasingly influential over the next few years
- **Conclusions and Questions** – points raised that may provoke further thinking

Lastly, in the appendix we have also included a summary of some of key insights gleaned from each workshop classified by location as well as associated rankings of many of the shared issues as judged by future potential impact.

As all our events are run under the Chatham House Rule,[2] we do not attribute quotes to any one individual or organisation. Instead we have sought to identify the discussions that insights were gleaned from. Therefore, throughout this document we have highlighted comments from the workshops in blue and also referenced key locations as appropriate.

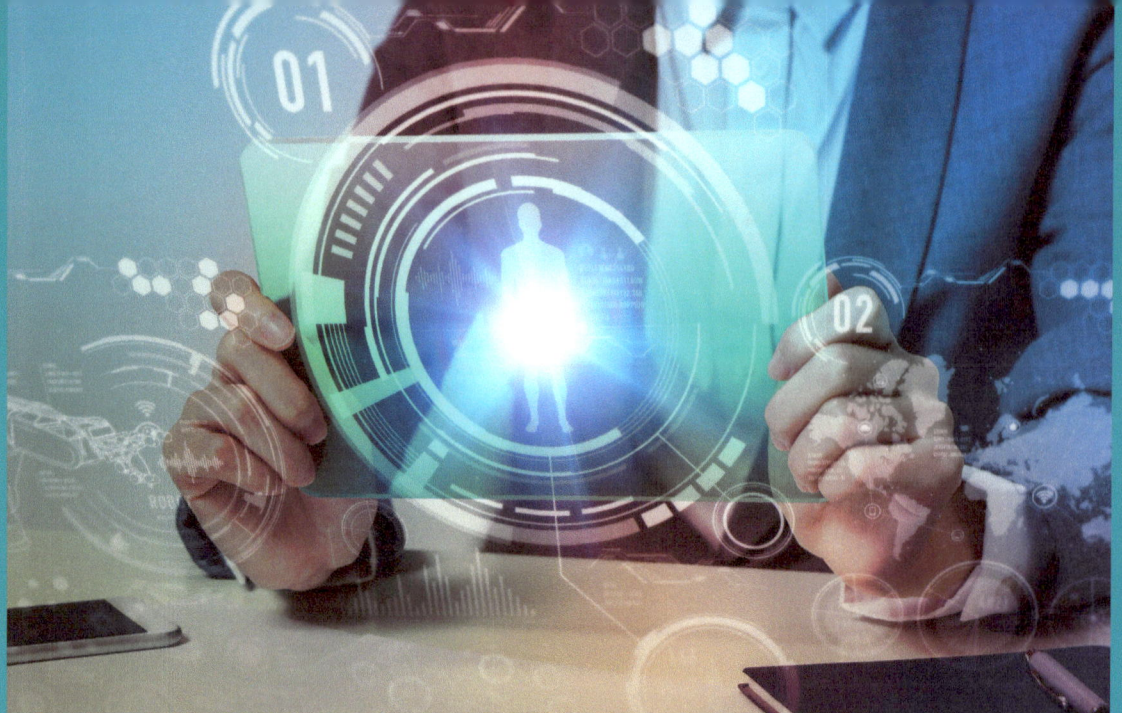

Context

Before delving into specific challenges and opportunities it is valuable to first replay views on some of the overall issues on both the future sources of patient data and some of the primary users of this information. In addition, we have highlighted the global ambitions for more and better use of patient data as an initial stake in the ground.

Sources of patient data

The patient data set is expanding: It includes high-quality clinical information, more personal data from apps and wearables, a broadening portfolio of proxy data as well as insights on the social determinants of health.

The increasing breadth of information available about our health is leading many to wonder what will constitute patient data in the future. The growing use of personal technologies has opened the door to the convergence of medical data about patients generated by healthcare providers with a plethora of non-medical, lifestyle related data, much of which is generated by the patient.

As shown in the graph below, some are predicting a 300% growth in healthcare data between 2017 and 2020. It is clear that Electronic Health Records (EHR) are no longer the only point of reference and we are entering a new era of health monitoring. However moving forward it will be important to clearly define who will have access to what information, when and how.

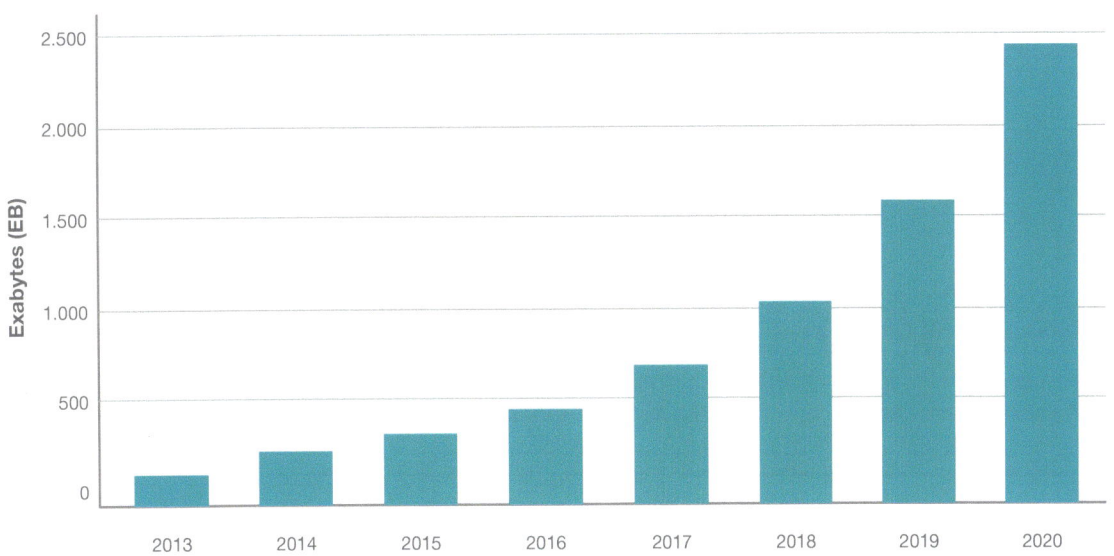

Growth In Healthcare Data

Source: EMC Digital Universe / IDC

To see the bigger picture about individuals' health we have to ensure that all data sources are recognized appropriately. While some medical data will remain rigorous and so potentially more reliable, many other sources of information could be useful if accessed, assessed and used in the right context. If an holistic approach is agreed, this allows a shift away from today's largely scientific / medically-oriented focus on illness towards one more concerned with staying well and which can include patient-generated, lifestyle related content. This approach will allow increased patient involvement in making informed decisions around the management of their own personal health care.

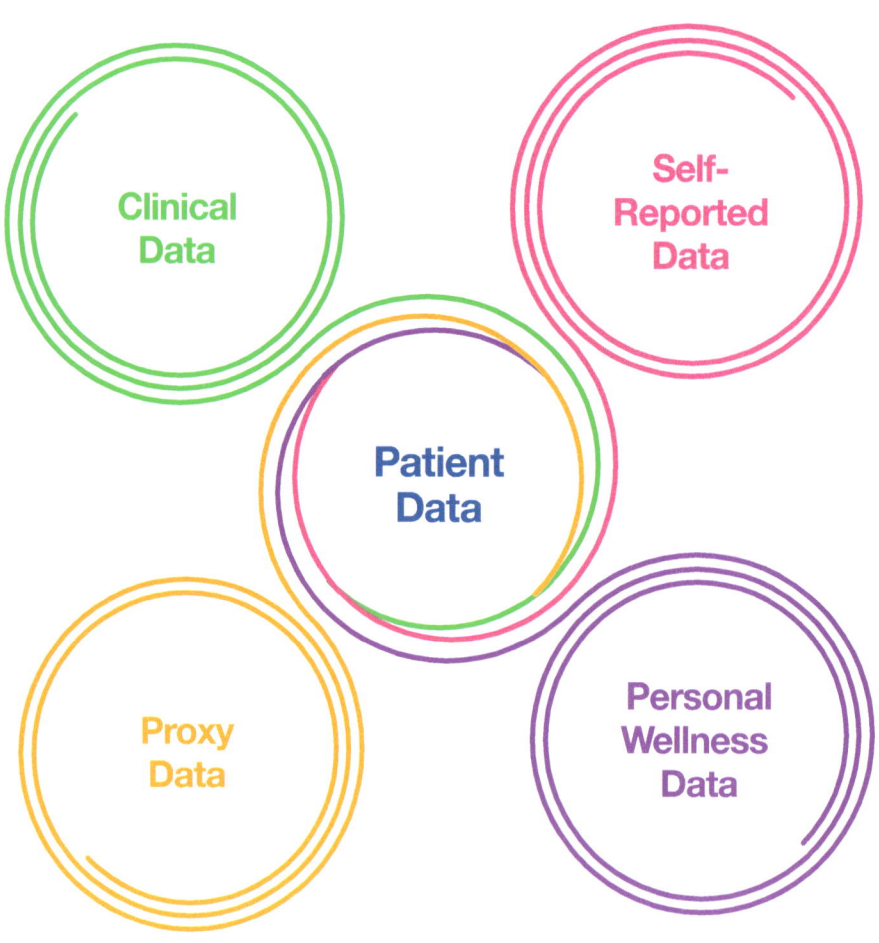

Alongside traditional data sets (e.g. clinical medical quality data typically found on the EHR; administrative data; claims information; health surveys; clinical trial results) we will expect to access other sources. These include:

- **Self-reported data** – such as blood pressure, heart rate, glucose levels, temperature, weight and in-home remote monitoring,

- **Personal wellness data** – such as feeds available from wearables, smart watches, fitness machines and numerous diet, exercise and social apps, and

- **Proxy data** – ranging from Facebook likes and Instagram comments to location and environmental data, resident post codes and even bathroom and fridge access

These are clearly not just patient-generated health data but also include a growing range of social-determinant information. As we gain access to additional contextual insight, there are a range of signals that can help build an accurate picture of the patient and his/her health.[3] However, having access to biometric, nutritional, clinical, fitness and even psychological information does not necessarily make it comprehensible. As was stated in Mumbai *"we are already data-rich but information-poor. Currently the data we have is not leveraged enough to help providers help patients."* It is clear we will also need better analytical tools to help make sense of the masses of additional material heading our way. *"Big data needs to be unlocked – the more organized we can get it, the more preventative we can be."*

There were several discussions around how proxy data is already providing additional insights on the social determinants of health. Lifestyle data is readily available through social media plus any number of fitness apps and devices. But there are many other opportunities to gather data which could be facilitated by technology and are currently available and under-utilized; for example, enabling delivery personnel to monitor and, importantly, report on any concerns they may have for the elderly or infirm they encounter as they carry out their rounds. In Boston the consensus was that new, efficient ways to collect data will change how ongoing healthcare support is provided. Different ways to observe eating habits were also discussed, such as by tracking when a fridge or oven door is opened. Equally 'gate detection' for repeated night-time bathroom access could act an early warning signal for possible UTI and so the need for increased care.

Looking ahead, many expect the increase in sensory monitoring to massively improve information capture from across the eco-system.[4] This is based on the assumption not only that the public will become less sensitive about sharing personal data but there will also be better analysis once more data is gathered. It also means we need to accommodate multi-dimensional data outside hospitals and so some big challenges will include managing not just the sheer volume of information but also identifying 'signal / noise ratios' that help us work out what is really important. Traditional population benchmarks, such as average life expectancy, may have to make way for new baselines for comparison; these could include a greater focus on years of active healthy ageing.

Users of patient data

The users and uses of the patient data set is broadening: Alongside the patient and traditional payers and providers it increasingly includes multiple new entrants seeking to disrupt and improve healthcare.

As well as a wider selection of sources of patient data, there is a correspondingly growing diversity amongst those who use, or plan to use, newly available individualized health information.

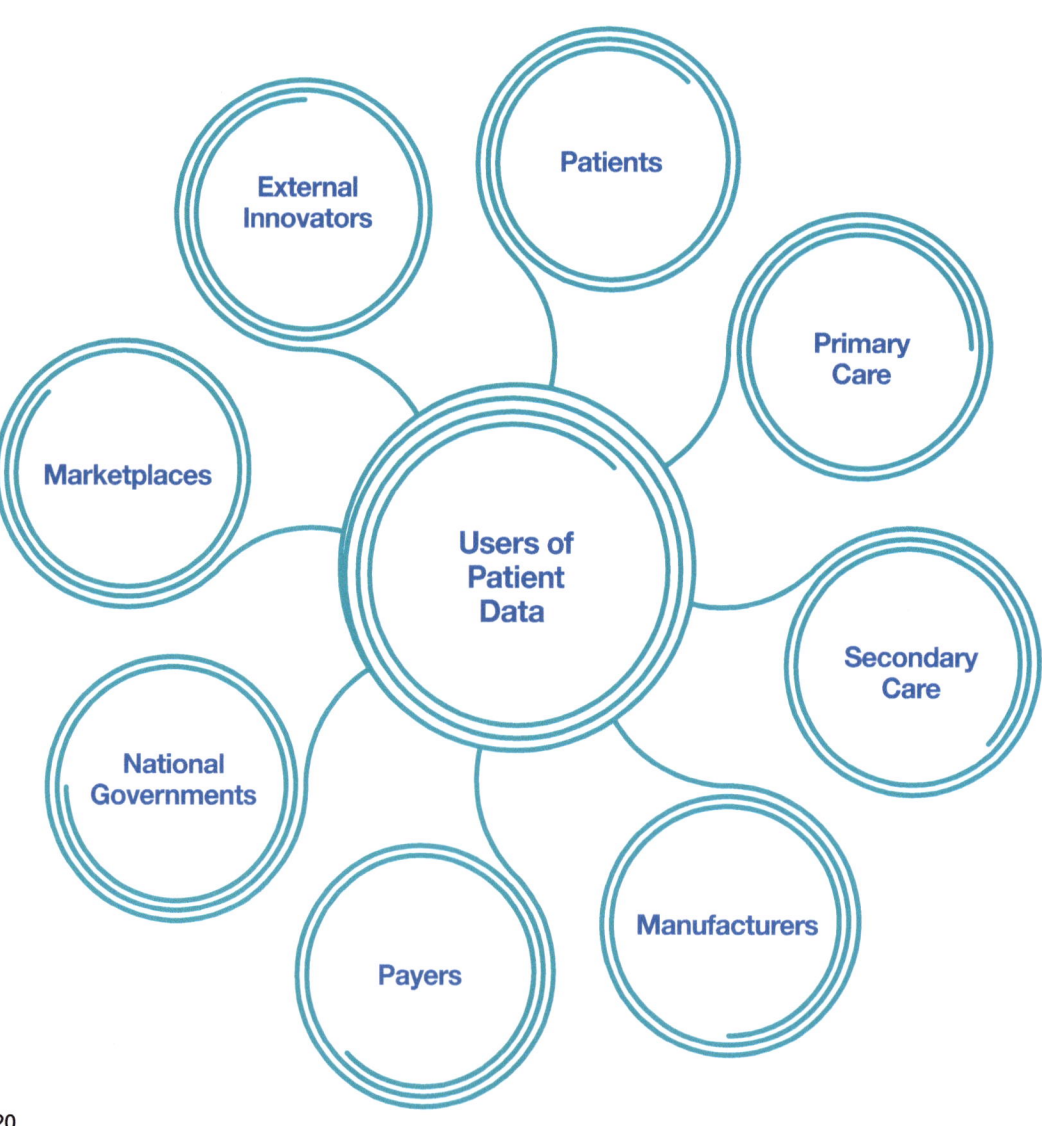

We have rapidly moved beyond just the traditional payer / provider portfolio to encompass a wider user-group, with new communities which, importantly, more frequently now include the patients themselves.[5] Across our global discussions, experts highlighted that going forward we should probably consider eight key user groups in terms of patient data access and use:

Patients – who are increasingly becoming better informed about their own health and fitness, as well as whether appropriate providers are accessing their data, when and why.

Primary Care - including GP practices, social care, pharmacies and community support all of whom want as much contextual insight as possible as well as quality health data to enable effective diagnosis and prescription.

Secondary Care – hospitals and clinics receiving patient metrics, scheduling appointments, providing remote support and running analytics on patient treatment and outcomes as well as integrating data within the EHR.

Manufacturers - such as medical device and pharmaceutical companies alongside associated service providers that want real-time analysis of performance, the ability to interrogate information to learn and refine their products.

Payers - including insurers, third-parties and health plan sponsors as well as, in many countries, government keen to track patient health, monitor interventions and reward successful outcomes.

National Governments – whether or not in single payer systems, national governments increasingly want to track individual and population wellness, so they can identify and manage risks to public health and national security.

Marketplaces – as health data is increasingly monetized and traded via new marketplaces, these markets themselves will need to be confident of the provenance and quality of the information as well as permissions to trade - even if the data is aggregated and anonymized.

External Innovators – big tech, start-ups and established IT companies all keen to improve the patient experience also require good-quality anonymized and aggregated data sets from patients to build, test and develop new services.

Recognizing not only these different potential users of patient data as groups, but also understanding their requirements for and use of data is critical. Although not all needs will be aligned all the time, harmonization and standardization of data to ensure high levels of use by all is clearly desirable.

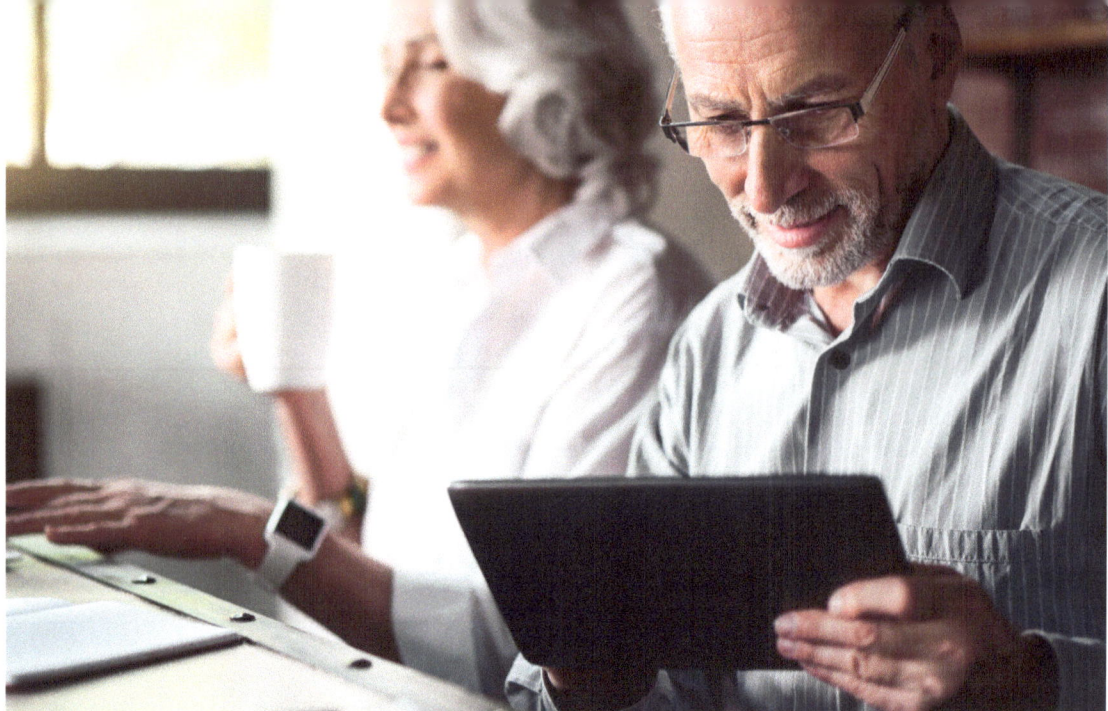

The global ambition

BENEFITS FOR THE PATIENT

Across all our discussions there was great anticipation of the benefits to be gained from access to more and better patient data. At its core, one common ambition is to 'give health data back to the individual' so that the patient becomes the point of integration and control. Patients will thus become more 'empowered' by having greater access to more information about their health and so will be able to make more informed decisions about their lifestyle choices. As more personal data will, in turn, enable more personalised healthcare so, the argument goes, this healthcare can become increasingly tailored to the individual – addressing their behavioural needs as well as their genetic predispositions. In this way there can be more accurate interventions and patients can be healthier for longer – a key benefit for an ageing population.

Richer data will open the door to more targeted responses facilitating predictive, personalized and effective healthcare. The advantage of this for a patient is that they can more easily see the potential benefit of preventative measures and therefore have a greater incentive to make timely behaviour changes. It could also mean that it will be easier to test and support more hypotheses prior to diagnosis.

If used in the right way data can also be a great communications tool and, as we collect more of it, it will become more precise in its ability to deliver relevant and targeted messages. There are already a number of successful initiatives including 'Stickk' for goal setting;[6] peer-based education, for instance NHS MMR vaccination stories; and agewell global[7] and Swordhealth[8] in Portugal where 3D sensors are providing real time feedback.

Most of those we consulted agreed that, if we are going to encourage people to more proactively engage in their health and related decisions, then more attention has to be focused on communicating the right information effectively and ensuring healthcare systems incorporate faster feedback from patients' data:[ix] *"We will need to have more compelling narratives to deliver and support behavioral and societal change."* We may, for example, seek to make more of positive feedback, such as Walgreen's success with using points as payback for drug compliance[10], rather than encourage negative pressures such as are generated by exercise monitors which highlight failure to meet set goals.[11] That said, in San Francisco it was pointed out that, we should be careful not to confuse consumers with patients. They are very different - *"consumers are increasingly digitally dependent, but patients are often digitally desperate."*

BENEFITS FOR THE SYSTEM

There are also wider benefits of access to better data – primarily for healthcare providers and payers who see the opportunity for far greater efficiency - especially in reducing complexity and improving compliance. At an industry level, richer data offers the opportunity for more experimentation to test then scale. More and better data about patient health will not only improve the effectiveness of individual healthcare but, by implication, at a population level enhance that of the whole health infrastructure. This is welcome news at a time when many healthcare systems are under increasing stress and ensuring that the benefits of this flow through is a priority for many. A recent Willis Towers Watson study found that U.S. employers expect their health care costs to increase by 5.5% in 2018, up from a 4.6% increase in 2017. The study projects an average national cost per employee of $12,850.[12] Getting this spend under better control is clearly a priority concern.

In principle creating and providing more health value for patients has always been both the ultimate goal and an increasingly critical competitive advantage for health care payers and providers worldwide. It is a continuous challenge, particularly when payer organisations are having to manage funding gaps and improve the care of members within a changing regulatory environment. Such are the growing pressures that many healthcare providers must transform their business models to deliver cost-competitive services that not only improve patient outcomes but are also expected to deliver sustainable growth for the organisation.[13] In many regions achieving this is about improving access. However, in nations where there is already pervasive healthcare, there are still constant demands for greater efficiency. Budgets are always tight and so any opportunity to improve efficiency is welcome.

The German and Swiss healthcare systems are often seen as the world's best[14] with the French method often in close contention.[15] However when *"value for money"* is considered, across Western nations, studies frequently identify the UK's NHS as the most efficient.[16] The US-based, Commonwealth Fund[17] analysis of healthcare systems in 11 nations finds NHS is the best, safest and most affordable.[18] Within this context, it was notable that in our London workshop it was suggested that *"many Western healthcare systems are on the verge of failing and without significant improvements in efficiency or major increases in funding they may collapse."* Better use of data is going to be pivotal. In US discussions the response was more prosaic, pointing out that healthcare systems have allegedly been on the edge of failure for decades, but they never do as 'customers' keep paying more. Indeed, in a New York discussion it was highlighted that, despite spending around 17% of GDP on healthcare, all expectations are that the money flow will continue to grow. That said, not everyone was optimistic, and another US opinion in Boston was that *"global healthcare is on the brink of a series of multiple systemic shocks that will force a rethink to a more efficient model – and this will apply across many nations - including the US".*

In Brussels, the assessment was that *"healthcare is struggling to manage budgets, but digitization provides an opportunity to identify the low-hanging fruit."* In London, it was seen that AI could be a key enabler of greater efficiency, while in Dubai it was envisaged that both AI and robotics will drive down healthcare costs: *"To deliver the envisioned change, massive parallel processing needs to take place - and this has to be aligned with much lower cost diagnostics across data sets. Only then can we achieve large-scale implementation that will provide cheaper, better diagnosis and start to have a positive impact on patients globally."*

The potential for greater efficiency was also highlighted elsewhere: *"Innovation happens when there are gaps and there are lots of gaps in India - so lots of opportunity."*[19] In South Africa, a major focus is the need to bridge the divide between the public and private systems. In Singapore, where there is increasing collaboration across multiple areas of activity, greater efficiency remains a core objective.

Our Toronto discussions highlighted the success of a system that has embraced evidence-based medicine where the focus is on the *"long run value"* of healthcare. Comparing the cost of prostate cancer treatment in Canada vs. the US was as a frequent reference point; in Canada it is limited to $6,500 per patient but in the US, it is much higher – over $30,000 in some cases. Another common issue raised in Europe is the need to improve end of life support.[20] Whether by more open discussion of palliative care, more data-enabled 'in-home' support or more transparent options for intensive care, refining the financial and social dimensions, is a growing priority.

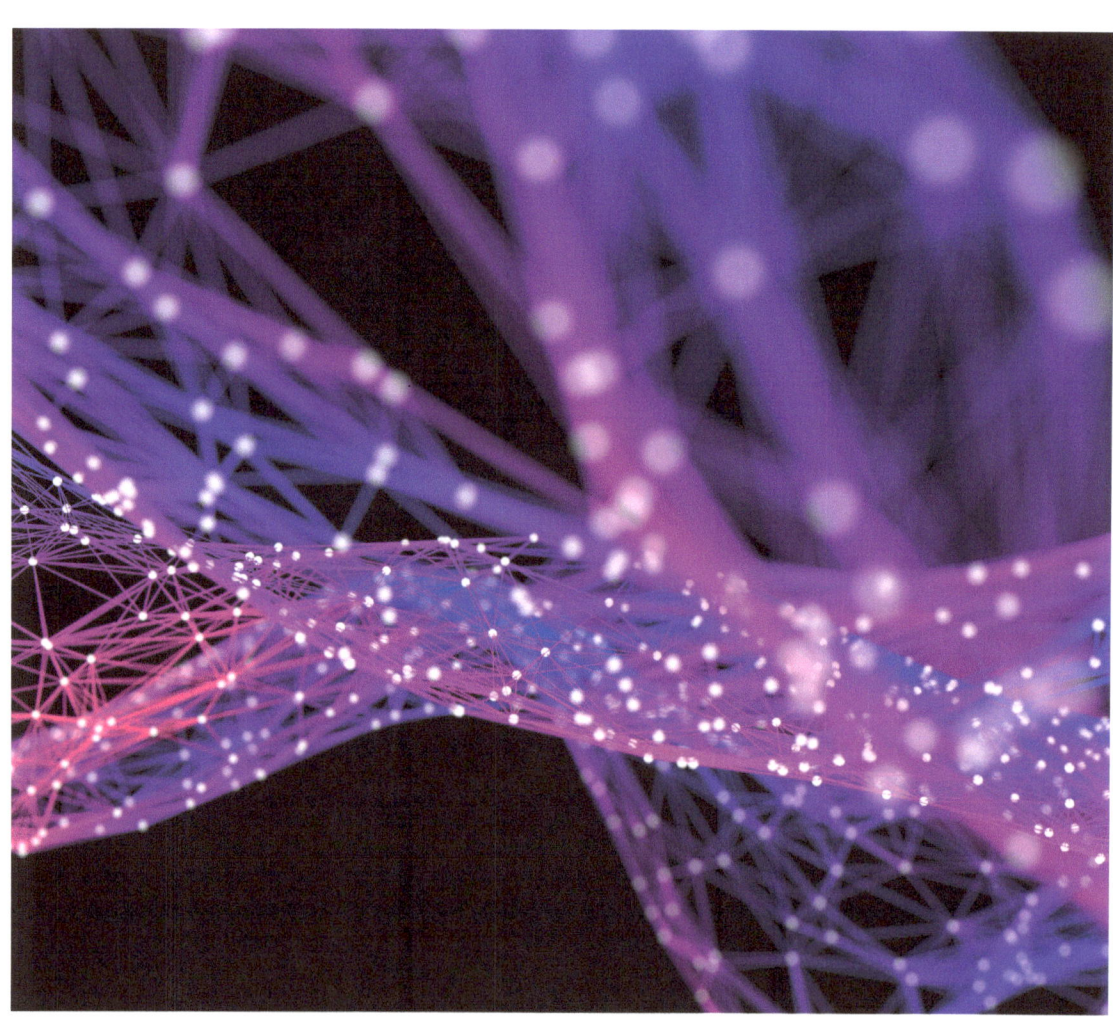

Unexpected outcomes

A number of experts also highlighted that there may also be a negative impact from too much data. A frequent concern in many foresight projects is that we do not think enough about the unexpected outcomes and unintended consequences of our well-intentioned actions.

In a previous programme exploring the future of food, a New York conversation highlighted the introduction of calories alongside prices on all restaurant menus. While designed to provide individuals with better information about the possible food options and so help people to make choices that improve their diet, this was not a universal outcome. Notably, for a good number of the urban poor, seeking to get value for money, the new menus allowed them to choose food options that provided the most calories per dollar. As such their behaviour was the opposite of what was intended.

Several experts in our discussions saw that there is often a downside about the growing dependence on technology. A question to consider therefore is what will be the unexpected outcome of all the new, more personalised information that is being generated, shared and analysed? For example, in the US and South Africa events there were comments from doctors about too much tech meaning that, *"we spend too much time looking at screens rather than patients' faces."*[21]

More accessible data, more accurate information and better analysis will, as we will see later, provide the opportunity for all to be healthier and receive better healthcare support – but it may, for instance, also result in the identification and exclusion from systems of those with very high or expensive health risks. As we embrace new technology and develop new models we should be cognizant of both risk and opportunity.

This will, we hope, help to support and validate many of the assumptions that you are making about how healthcare will improve over the next ten years. In addition, as it shares a broad range of views drawn from many different expert voices around the world, it may also challenge some of your current perspectives and lead to new opportunities for innovation in and around patient data. We hope that it is a useful addition to your library.

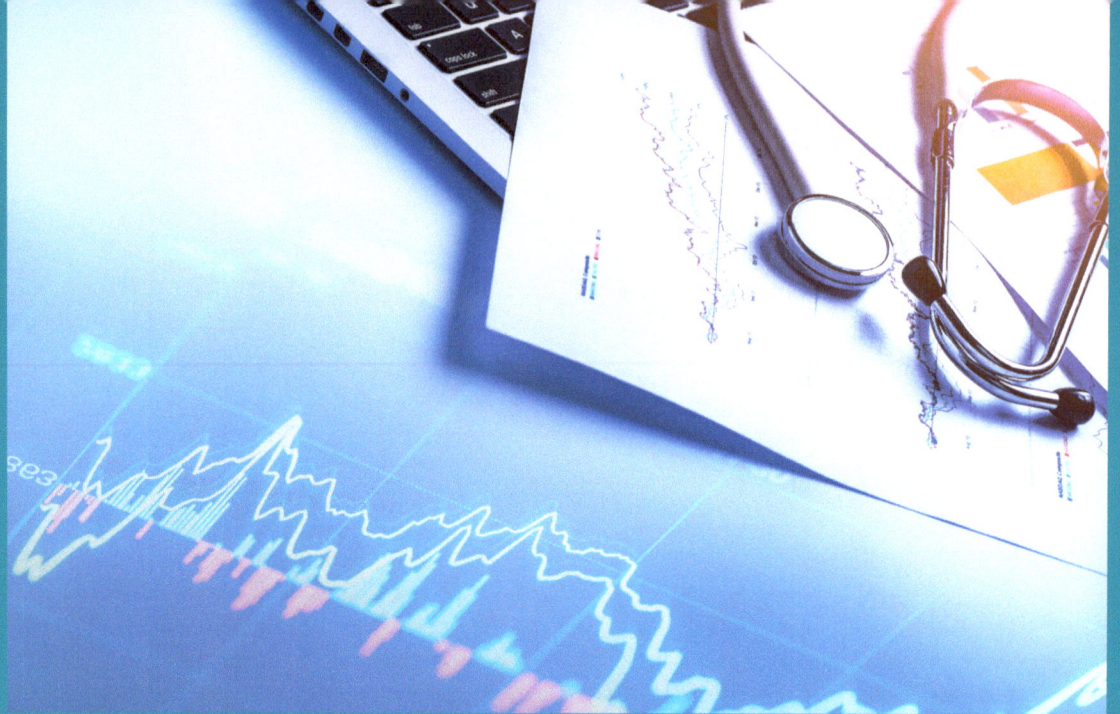

Shared challenges

Across our varied discussions there were a number of issues that are often seen as common challenges. While the specific nuance may vary by region and stakeholder, these are all viewed as obstacles to be overcome. Indeed, without successfully addressing them, many felt that the wider ambitions for and opportunities from better use of patient data may well be difficult to achieve. As such, these shared challenges appear to be a current priority for many.

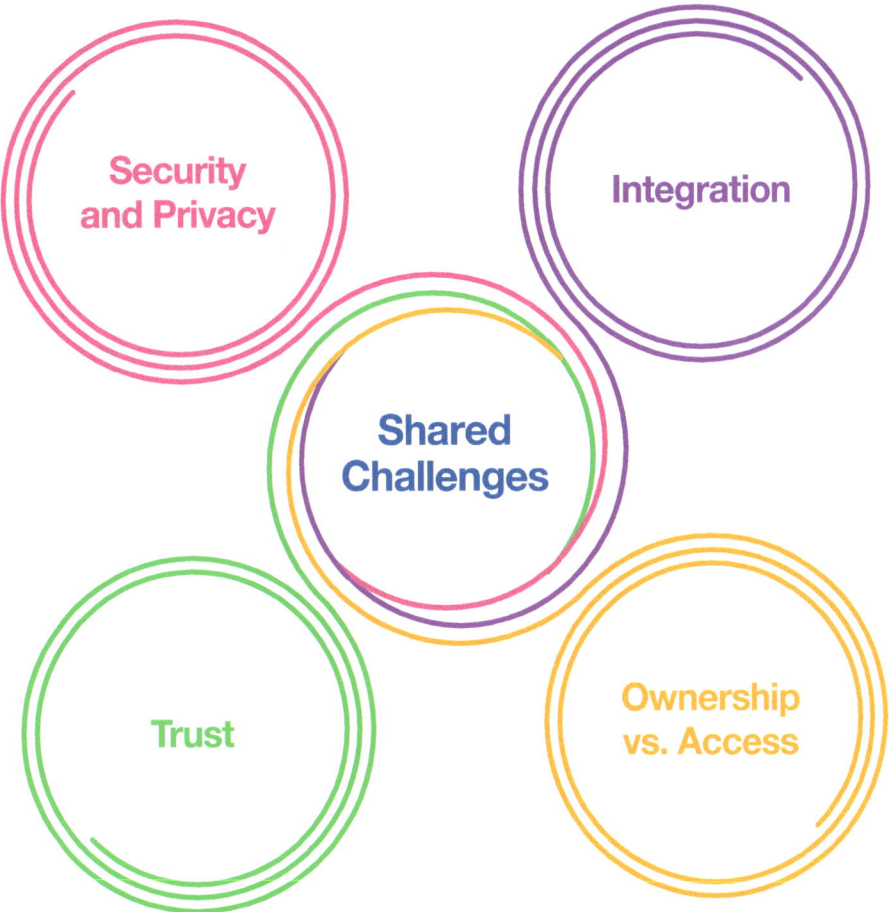

Integration – Although some organisations are wary of sharing valued information, several governments and markets seek new ways to merge disparate data sets for greater social benefit. As the appetite to scale and combine new sources of personal, societal and clinical information increases, the expectation is that technology will provide solutions that better bridge data gaps and ensure inter-operability in the future. Establishing common standards across data sets will be a key driver of change.

Trust – In many regions, trust needs to be (re)built between payers, providers and patients as well as with new entrants coming into the healthcare arena. New technology platforms and improving communication with the public both play a major role. Concern about ulterior motives for the use of data is high and some see AI adding to the challenge. Many recognise the need for greater transparency on practice in some pivotal areas.

Ownership vs. Access – If access to patient data is to have impact it needs to be aggregated and shared but there are concerns around ownership and who makes decisions around its use. Patients may have increasing control of their data, but whether they are its real custodians and are able to control access to it depends on culture, regulation and need. Many countries are moving towards supporting greater individual access and ownership of health data – a question will be how well citizens engage with it.

Security and Privacy – As anonymized, aggregated data is more easily re-linked and sensitive health data is a target for cyber-attacks, questions are raised around the benefits of centralized vs. decentralized data and the impact of localization. Given both the sensitivity and value of healthcare data it is little surprise that security and privacy are high on multiple agendas. As vulnerability and risk increase apace with greater focus from external hackers and internal sources, these are growing concerns for many.

Each are detailed in the following pages

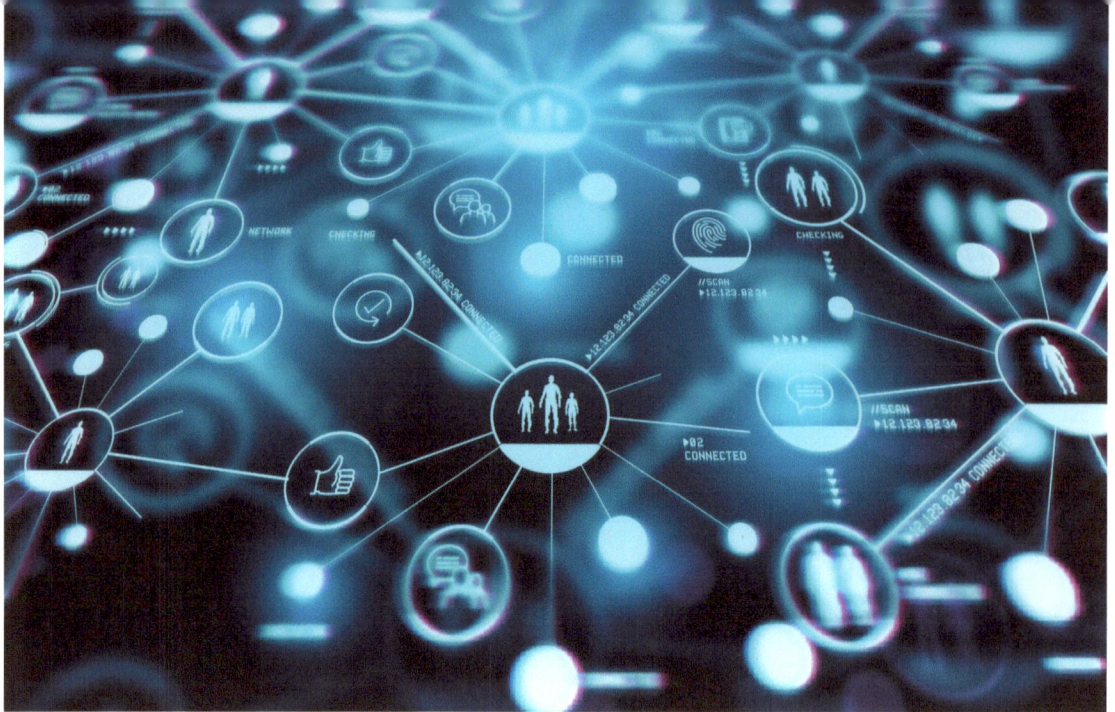

Integration

Although some organisations are wary of sharing valued information, several governments and markets seek new ways to merge disparate data sets for greater social benefit. As the appetite to scale and combine new sources of personal, societal and clinical information increases, the expectation is that technology will provide solutions that better bridge data gaps and ensure interoperability in the future. Establishing common standards across data sets will be a key driver of change

Although there has been a proliferation of health data and its collection, many see that we are not yet at a point of unleashing its power because the vast majority of information remains proprietary and fragmented among insurers, providers, health record companies, government agencies, and researchers. Despite the technological integration seen in banking and other industries, healthcare data has largely remained scattered and inaccessible.[22] Indeed attempts to make hospitals and clinics more efficient by building huge, centralized IT systems have a sorry history - just look at a failed patient-record system for Britain's National Health Service, scrapped after 10 years at a cost of around £10 billion ($15 billion).

BARRIERS

Part of the difficulty is that many of today's healthcare systems are rife with multiple and legacy systems. In the US, for example, EHRs currently remain fragmented among 860 ambulatory care vendors and 270 in patient vendors. Others are similarly disjointed. IT issues such as compatibility and version control are obvious hurdles, as is the fact that many healthcare systems are increasingly strapped for cash, which inhibits their ability to secure sustained financial support for the investment required. At some point the nettle will have to be grasped and significant investments made.

To date the global healthcare industry has largely struggled to successfully manage the myriad stakeholders, regulations, and privacy concerns required to build a fully integrated healthcare IT system.[23] The problem is clear; the Institute of Medicine sees that: *"A significant challenge to progress resides in the barriers and restrictions that derive from the treatment of medical care data as a proprietary commodity by the organisations involved… Broader access and use of healthcare data for new insights require not only fostering data system reliability and interoperability but also addressing the matter of individual data ownership and the extent to which data central to progress in health and health care should constitute a public good."*[24]

NOT SHARING

It is true that many organisations see that their data has both commercial and competitive value so the principle of sharing this more freely is not an easy conversation to have. Currently several major healthcare organisations do not share their data and see no benefit in changing, *"not with Google nor with Apple even though they are asking for it: Partly this is about ethics but also about ownership and use."* In addition to this some are wary of providing international access to patient data because of security concerns. With the rising tide of data hacks and wider cyber-security now a mainstream concern in healthcare, the idea of centralized ownership of medical records is increasingly being viewed by some as a security risk. They argue that *"we need to decentralize this data because the more it's amassed, the more likely it's going to be hacked."* Better regulation may go some way to address this conundrum and indeed a number of guidelines are being shared which set standards, but, as yet, there are few incentives for organisations or nations to deliver. Also, aside from the security and ethical issues many point out that standardizing data from the current disparate data sets is an expensive and time-consuming business. And no one has yet answered the fundamental question of *"who will pay money to clean data."*[25]

CONNECTING DATA

The technological difficulties of combining disparate sources of information into a commonly accessible format should not be underestimated. There is certainly great hope that it can be achieved with multiple organisations and governments, many under pressure from escalating costs, aspiring to an end-point where the entirety of an individual's health data is clearly presented, easily accessed, available for analysis and, at the same time, protected. Realistically this possibility, even for sophisticated healthcare services, is a few years or so away. A good number of organisations expect to be grappling with legacy systems, poor interoperability and unstructured data for quite some time to come. In the short term the ambition for many is therefore to achieve better connectivity between data sets within the clinical arena by improving harmonization, standardisation and data quality.

Beyond this there is growing recognition of the value of self-generated personal and proxy data. Although this is often more unstructured and does not meet current medical standards, it does provide a contextual richness for clinicians which helps them to better understand patient health. Many agree that more rigorous collection and analysis of this will be of great benefit and will help to shift healthcare away from treatment of conditions to one that prevents illness, *"today we have 1% wellness data and 99% clinical – in future it will be 99% wellness and 1% clinical."*

What is clear is that there is *"a tsunami of health data heading our way"* and making the best out of this relies on the ability to integrate the most useful information and make it more widely accessible. Many agree that we are generating more data than we can currently use and expect the situation will continue simply because of the impending *"data storm of information coming from millions of people."*

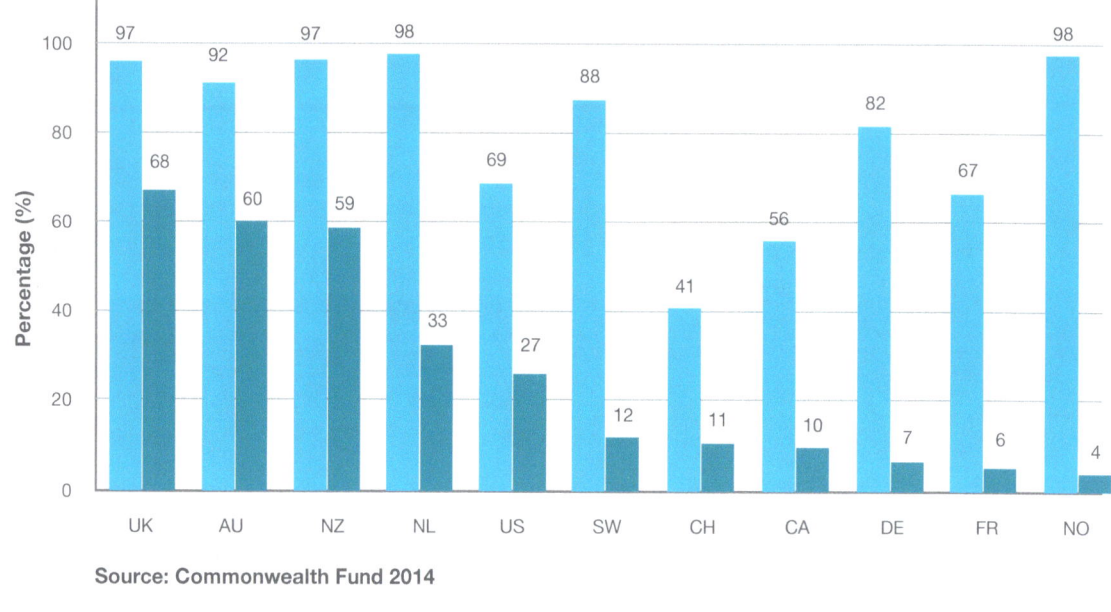

Doctors with EHR and Multifunctional Health IT Capacity

Source: Commonwealth Fund 2014

● Uses EHR   ● Uses EHR with multifunctional HIT capacity

In Oslo, however, the view was that managing this is a temporary challenge and that by 2030 *"there will be no real barriers to combining both structured and unstructured data. There will be better quality of data, more standardization and greater harmonization."* Others were keen to point out that *"healthcare is a multi-disciplinary team sport and we need to be able to share and use insights and information more smoothly and effectively – and see the bigger picture not just a silo."*[26]

STANDARDISATION

Quite how this ambition can be achieved given the highly fragmented systems found in many countries today is not obvious. Already boasting a high-quality healthcare service, Singapore is making strong moves around multi-data set connectivity, but other countries are facing much more fundamental challenges. Irrespective of location, most workshop participants agreed that, in order to take advantage of new technologies, strategies must be developed that will align regulation, funding models and outcome-based incentives. Once a common framework is developed, the notion of a connected information set that could act as a 'personal health passport' becomes more realistic. At the moment this is the long-view, even for Singapore where our discussion focused primarily on the need for greater institutional sharing of data between government departments such as the ministries of social development, health and education. Looking ahead the ambition is that, *"by 2030, payers (both private and public) will use standardized platforms to produce and consume data. Moreover, patients will be incentivized to bring in their own data sets for aggregation to improve the ease of access to services."*

Given all this, what then are some specific technological challenges that need to be addressed?

CLEAN DATA

Data is only useful if it is clean, structured and has context. However, often the quality of the health data available is insufficient for many clinical services

– and as one workshop participant observed *"garbage in means garbage out."* In order to gain cleaner data *"we need a common language between all stakeholders."* Several believe that *"the current system does not encourage this. In fact, it incentivises the reverse. As a result, there isn't much communication between specialists, hospitals and GPs."* Furthermore, there is currently very little consistency around how data is collected; notes are written in one surgery which may not be recognized in another thus making it problematic for anyone to manage the transfer of information between doctors. On top of this it is sometimes difficult to ascertain which organisation generated what information in the first place so how to agree who may be reasonably considered responsible for updating and maintaining its quality is almost impossible. This becomes even more complex when you consider that often data is co-created – and then shared. Some see that there has to be a universal agreement to improve standards but at the moment *"even the FDA is struggling to decide what data has to be cleaned."* Moreover, as shown in the graph below, although there has been a rise in the number of doctors using EHRs, those using HER with multifunctional capacity are, in many countries, still low.

CLASSIFIED DATA

Another important issue is how to manage the combination of high quality medical information with lower quality personal data as well as all the potential proxy data. Present standards around consumer generated data do not meet the higher medical quality thresholds. Many are concerned. *"How do we know what good data is when we are mixing professional information with passive (consumer) data?"* In particular *"Fit-bit data has to have more relevance to make it worthwhile - wearables are not providing medical standard data and so we need to work hard to raise the standards"* and *"there is growing interest in helping consumer generated data to meet medical grade quality levels."*

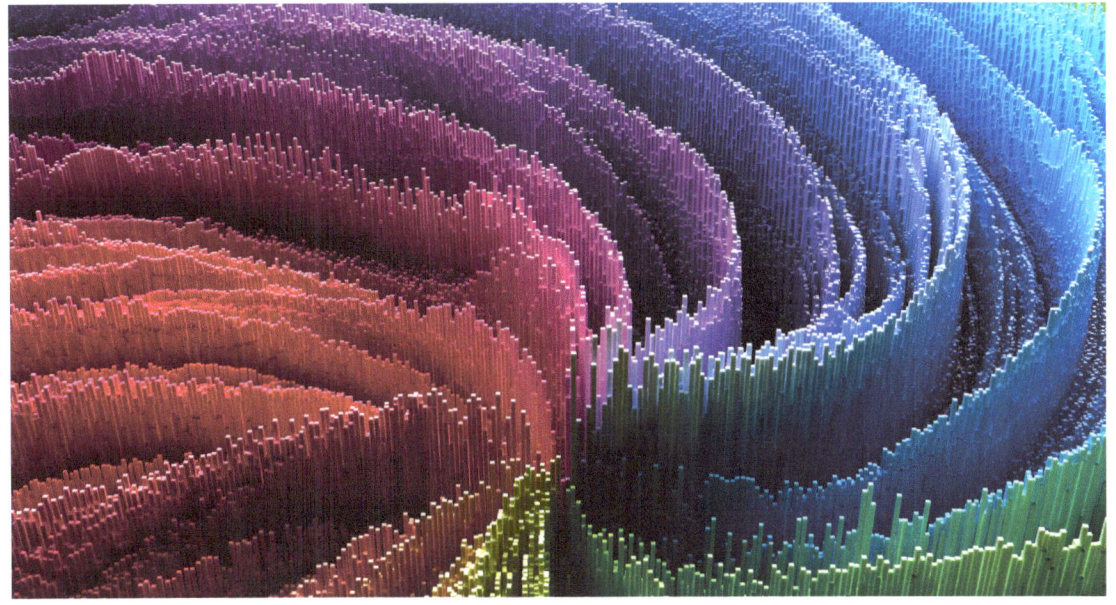

However, just because data is not of medical quality does not mean it has no value. It's all a question of what information is appropriate. Sometimes *"the data that someone is wearing a fit-bit is itself very valuable and insightful"* – it may be poor quality, but it is a good proxy for healthy activity: *"Who cares about the information quality when we know that someone cares enough about their health to wear a fit-bit?"* Self-reported population data also has great empirical value. *"As long as we know what data we are mixing and can classify it accordingly then we can make good use of the information."* To be useful, some argued, data has to be 'good enough' not always of the highest quality. In San Francisco, the suggestion was that better data classification will provide insight between high value, low value and peripheral information. This reinterprets the challenges to be less about cleaning data and more about how best to combine different quality data sets and use it appropriately: "We have to integrate direct and indirect data." Clearly issues around broader data gaps need to be solved so that it is possible to *"marry up non-traditional data (e.g. weather patterns, air quality, location of parks etc.) with health data"* to better understand patient needs.

INTEROPERABILITY

Many would say that combining datasets has really only ever worked in fairly simple cases with small populations and with relatively few interconnections. With systems as widely varying and disparate as those found across the healthcare sector, it could well be that immense, centralized systems will never completely offer efficient platforms as there are just too many moving parts. Picking the data worth sharing and matching it with the most appropriate platforms around specific issues, conditions, demographics or public vs. private healthcare systems is seen by many as the most pragmatic approach. All the same, most advocate the need for better interoperability, to enable different information technology systems and software applications to communicate, exchange data, and then put the information that has been exchanged to effective use. *"Closing the information loop will foster interoperability and motivate participants to make better use of data."*

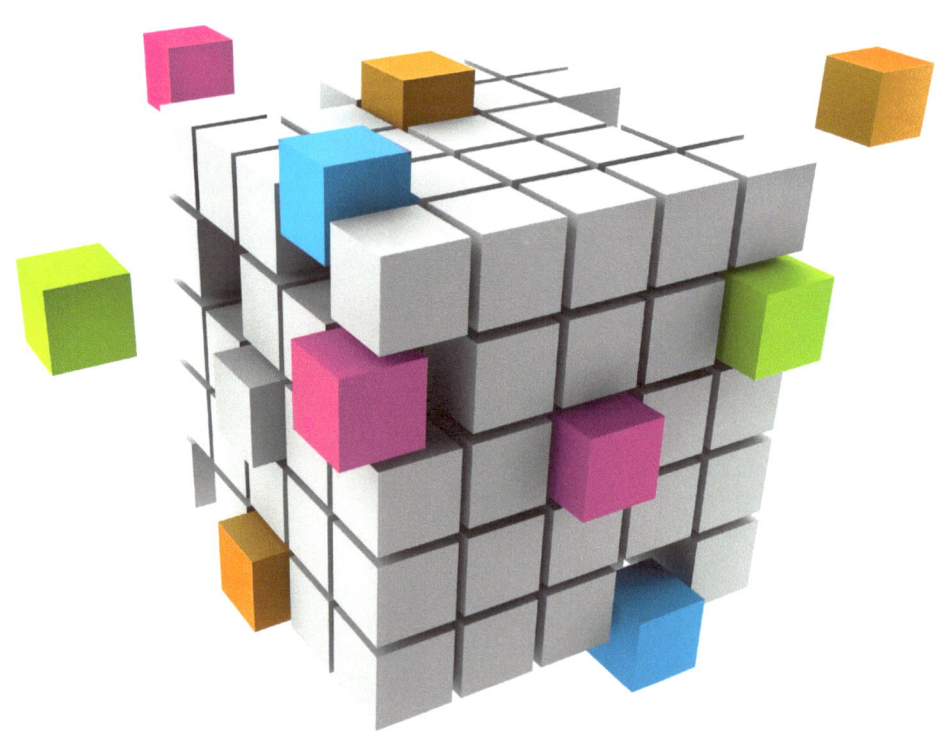

THE ROLE OF POLICY

If, as some suggest, we are moving towards universal healthcare data access then we will create a world where information silos are connected, probably via third parties which are able to unify, mine and discover new insights. To do this we will not only have to solve the technological challenge but crack a range of complex ethical and commercial issues as well. Across Europe, despite common ambitions, it was felt that current regulation is preventing progress: *"It's all about interfaces but there is no shared understanding, particularly regionally."* Addressing this is fundamental to the progress of data use within the healthcare system and many felt that *"technically it's not a challenge but policy makers need to step up."*

Beyond political will, some major steps for government-led change include addressing the technological difficulties involved in dealing with centralized and de-centralized interoperability, improving analytics (which varied governments will support to ensure and track standards of care as well as risk stratification) and driving the systems towards better care efficiencies.

It seems clear that as patients and doctors grow more used to new technologies there will be further collaboration across healthcare. *"Getting to an outcome-based system will require a more open market with socially beneficial products utilizing the data aligning with top down government funded activities to build trust."* However, establishing trust in the system will be a long road and not all countries will have the public support nor the technical ability to achieve this for some time. One of the regulatory sticking points, for example, is how to identify an effective way of managing patient consent. Ultimately most believe that necessity will mean that global standards will eventually be created but it will take time; even garnering local agreement in Europe is difficult; America has a different approach; China and India, both of which have more people online than Europe and America have citizens, have another.

AN INTEGRATED SYSTEM

Everyone wants a system where the patient is both active and aware of their involvement in their own care. Several examples of progress, good and bad were cited. In both Oslo and London, the UK care.data approach[27] was mentioned as a failed endeavour – especially concerning the sharing of sensitive medical information with commercial companies without the explicit consent of patients.[28] However the Swiss hybrid model for healthcare[29] was well regarded. Moving forward it is agreed that within Europe there is a lot of positive focus on creating a federation of databases but in doing so we should adopt the FAIR data principles – where Findability, Accessibility, Interoperability and Reusability are all at the core.[30] In the US it is suggested that in order to create the right regulatory environment, it is important to consider *"how to move beyond data harvesting to actually achieving something with the data."*

Within this a number of organisations are seeking to lead change. Companies such as **Validic** (see case study) have already started to combine multiple sources of personal data into one platform that can then be linked to an individual's medical records via the EHR. However meaningfully adding and matching in other proxy data is adding extra complexity. Part of the attraction of organisations such as **Flatiron Health** (see case study) is that they are taking a mass of unstructured data and using expert human input are curating it into a more coherent form for sharing and analysis.

As discussed in more detail later, there are clearly high expectations about the role that varied elements of AI can play in helping with better data integration. However, while some are focused on the longer-term future where the deep learning may better have the capability to deal with unstructured data, for now, many recognise that the first phases of AI application, focused on machine learning and pattern recognition, requires good quality structured data to interrogate. Consequently, there are a wealth of start-ups and new partnerships with the likes of GE, Google, Microsoft and IBM all seeking to help with this data cleaning and structuring.[31]

Perhaps the most notable recent move is however that of **Apple** (see case study) which sees healthcare as a major future area of focus. Given its long-term stance of 'differential privacy' and not extracting value for its customers' encrypted data, the company has now changed its position. In January 2018, after three years of preparing its devices to process medical data, Apple released its updated Health App which has raised the game. Users can now transfer clinical data direct from health providers to their iPhones, sharing the same information with their doctors. The aim is to provide as much transparency and long-terms visibility for personal health information as is available for financial data.[32]

Benefits for the Patient

It is only by having all the varied sources of personal health information effectively joined up that the promise of better use of patient data can be fulfilled. Integration is therefore clearly fundamental to the future ambition. If all of an individual's health records, personal wellness data as well as important proxy data can, indeed, be both co-located and combined, then this is what will open the door to the much-improved analysis, diagnosis and support that all are seeking.

CASE STUDY:

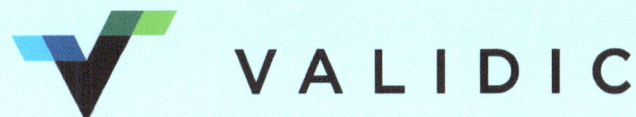

Founded in 2010, US based Validic has become one of the healthcare industry's leading technology platforms for convenient, easy access to digital health data from 'best-in-class' clinical sources. The company has to date raised more than $18 million, much of which came from Kaiser Permanente's venture capital arm. It doesn't monitor patients itself. Rather, it acts as a conduit and dashboard for all the inconsistent data streams emanating from various mobile health and in-home devices, fitness equipment, clinical sensors, activity wearables, smart bands and wellness applications: Information that would otherwise be impossible for doctors and health systems to keep up with and compare.[33] It is providing a one-stop source of much of the non-clinical sources of information that are increasingly part of the patient data mix.

At its core the company is in what it calls the 'conversation economy' which is moving across from social networks into healthcare and helping to provide 'participant-generated data.' "Patients today are expecting more than just episodic care transactions; they're behaving like consumers and want personalized, easy interactions with providers."[34] As such it is focused on improving user engagement through machine learning and seeking to curate a holistic view of wellness.[35] This is important because, as part of the combination, Validic takes data from legacy medical devices that are not even connected to the internet such as a traditional blood pressure cuff. It does this by encouraging patients to take a picture of the reading on their smartphone. For many of the companies that take the output, key issues are simplification, standardization and the means by which to start new conversations with patients. Organisations from hospitals and IT companies to pharma, insurance and health device manufacturers are all customers. So, companies such as Philips integrate the consumer-generated health data from Validic into their own digital platforms that in turn underpin the Philips connected health solutions and services.[36] Moving ahead, the aim is that, as remote monitoring and analytics technologies evolve, the company can provide much more of the increasing portfolio of important health data that is not on the core EHR.[37]

CASE STUDY:

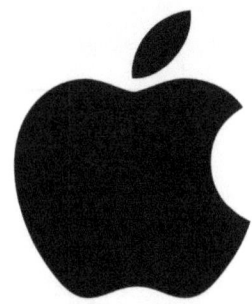

It is little surprise that the world's most valuable tech company has health data ambitions. Although one of the most secretive of the big tech firms, especially concerning long-term aims, some of its digital health ambitions are starting to emerge.[38] After a 'soft-entry' into the market in 2014 with the release of the Health App, the next layer occurred 12 months later with the launch of ResearchKit and the Apple Watch. Since then the company has rapidly built a platform for health data. Apple CEO Tim Cook sees that "health care is big for Apple's future."

Commentators have seen that Apple has several opportunities to exploit.[39] These include:

- Revenues with so much cash that, unlike many others, it is not dependent on insurers' reimbursement.

- Starting with Apple Watch fitness data, an acquisition of Gliimpse[40] (which lets users gather health information from disparate sources and share it with the healthcare institutions) and partnership with Health Gorilla, the company is gaining the clinical-grade data to offer a full personal health record.

- ResearchKit is a platform for large-scale research studies, streamlining the on-boarding process, that has changed the scale at which studies are done and the type of data that can be captured.

- The company has also been involved in diabetes and heart disease-management, connecting patients to the care they need when they need it via partnerships with American Well and others.

In January 2018, after three years of preparing its devices to process medical data, Apple released its updated Health App which has raised the game. Users can now transfer clinical data direct from health providers to their iPhones, sharing the same information with their doctors. The aim is to provide as much transparency and long-terms visibility for personal health information as is available for financial data.[41] The updated Health Records section within the Health app brings together hospitals' and clinics' information to make it easy for consumers to see their available medical data from multiple providers whenever they choose.[42]

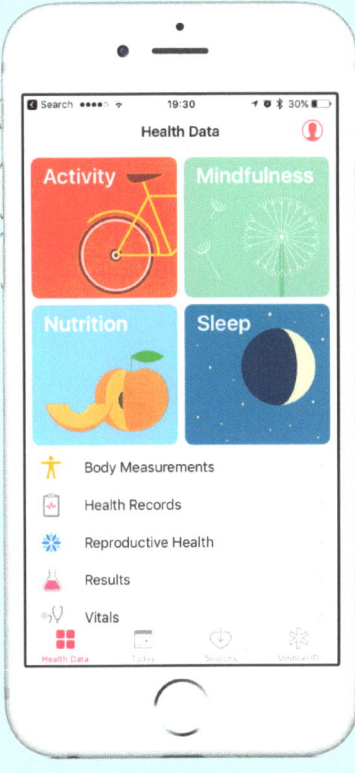
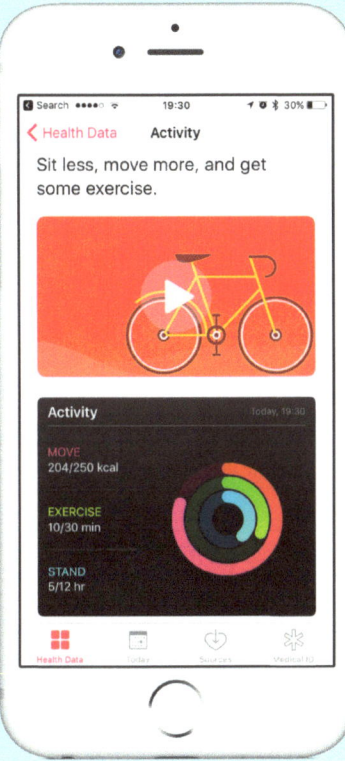
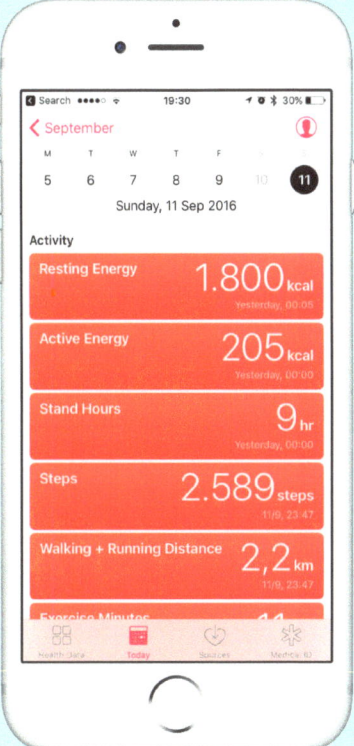

However, in a notable departure from its 'we will not see your data' policy due to encryption on the device, Apple now has the caveat for 'users to choose to share it with the company'. For a firm that has previously focused on devices and not data, this signals a potential major shift in future direction. While having the most trusted products through which medical data can flow is still the core priority for growing its core consumer base, the data business is now in play.[43] With the recent recruitment of a wealth of health, biotech and biomedical talent, the ability to embed the next generation of sensors within all its products to generate, capture and analyse more personal health data.

Apple has patents to turn its phones in full medical devices using new sensors to measure blood pressure, body fat and heart function. Equally its headphones are poised to undertake biometric monitoring and the Apple Watch is tracking blood glucose levels and heart health.[44] Furthermore, new apps are coming on line with at least 150 firms globally now developing some form of what have been termed 'digital therapeutics'.[45] At heart, a long-game approach with patients as consumers at the centre seems to fit with Apple's style.[46]

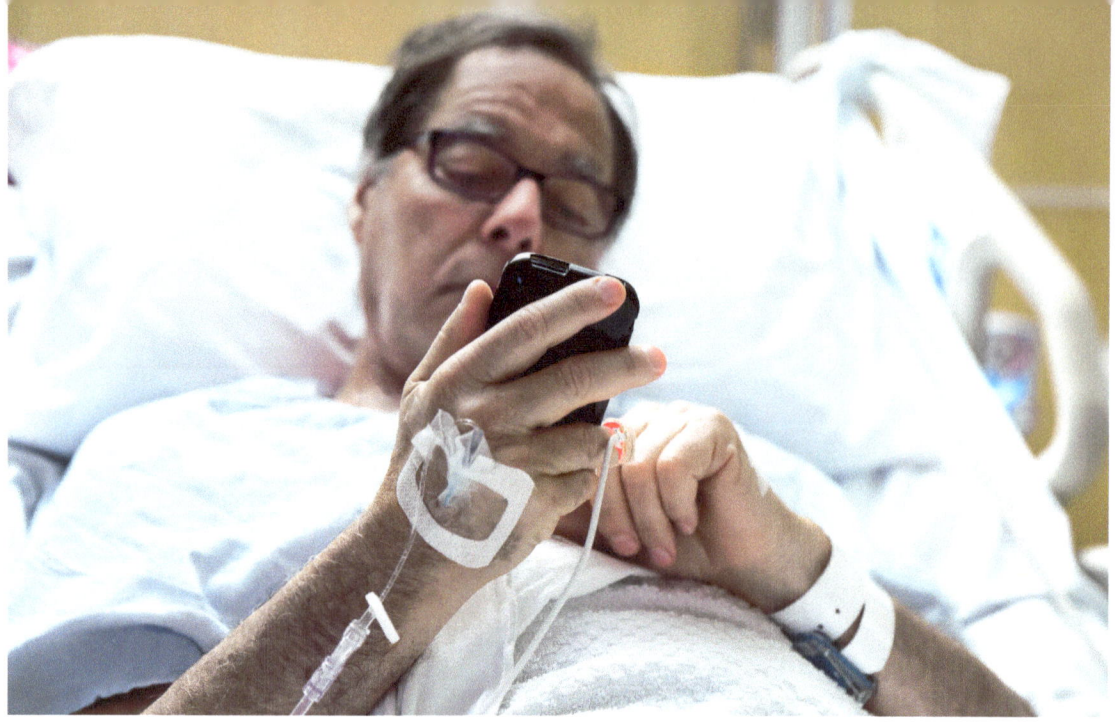

Ownership vs. access

If access to patient data is to have impact it needs to be aggregated and shared but there are concerns around ownership and who makes decisions around its use. Patients may have increasing control of their data, but whether they are its real custodians and are able to control access to it depends on culture, regulation and need. Many countries are moving towards supporting greater individual access and ownership of health data – a question will be how well citizens engage with it.

Everyone is talking about the importance of sharing data but the current ambiguities around how this can be done is proving to be a real barrier. As expectations are growing it is becoming increasingly important to understand who should own health data, who should control it and therefore who should best be able to make decisions around its access and use.

Some believe that ultimate ownership of health records should belong to the individual. After all who else will consider it important to keep that their health records are kept up to date? This is particularly relevant as health data is now being generated on personal devices - pretty much anyone can already take unlimited blood pressures or blood glucose measurements via a smartphone and choose whether or not to share the results.

So why not extend that decision-making ability to other aspects of their health data? But others point out that although organisations and healthcare professionals understand how, where and why to use new sources of data, it doesn't necessarily mean that patients will comprehend what could be the implication of what they choose to share. This might limit their ability to make the right choice about the use of their own records. Also, although the 'informed healthy' and 'worried well' may have good comprehension of what the data is saying, in many regions, concerns were raised about the ability of the 'average patient' or one in acute need or stress to be able to access and control the flow of information necessary for their own care.

REGAINING CONTROL

Although individuals may not fully understand how to control their digital footprints, one thing for sure is that they are increasingly distrustful of some third-party providers that are often in charge of access today. As we become more aware of the way personal data has been used, sold, repackaged and resold, there is a growing swell of public distrust in the current system which allows corporates to hold and capitalize on the use of personal information from the myriad sources they have access to. Not only does this already feel like an unnecessary personal intrusion for some, but many agree that the ways some data is currently stored and shared dramatically increases the risk of privacy breaches. This is either through the deliberate re-selling without permission or unintentionally, because of poor security and the escalation of cyber-attacks. It also raises questions about the need to better regulate the business models - sometimes termed *"surveillance capitalism"* because of their dependence on the sale and resale of personal data. Small surprise, perhaps, why some argue that the only way of regaining control of the situation, certainly for health data, is to ensure that data ownership remains in the hands of the individual who generated it. Whether that is more secure is currently an open question for some. However, looking ahead many believe the patient will not only have access to their own data, but they will increasingly also own it and control it, choosing how it can be shared and with which organisations.

OWNERSHIP

The challenge however is to build consensus around how to achieve this and then how to reasonably manage access data. Currently there seem to be more problems than answers. These were just some questions raised during our workshops:

- Who is responsible and accountable for the creation, upkeep and sharing of associated information?

- Who owns the data today?

- There will be a massive increase in the amount of data, but will ownership also increase?

- All US medical visits are captured electronically, and the data can now be combined – but if this happens who will be in control and manage this?

- How will individuals take ownership?

- What are the costs?

- What about policy impact?

- Once the information is collated, does this actually give individuals improved awareness, and will people better understand their own health risk?

Such is the ambiguity around the issue that there are many approaches around ownership models currently in play even within a single market. For example, in the US the Health Insurance Portability and Accountability Act (HIPAA) does not specify ownership, and state laws are inconsistent. For instance, only New Hampshire has a law which specifically states that patients own their medical records. Legal opinion ranges widely from *"the general understanding of the legal community is that patients own their records, or it's their interests that are ultimately paramount"* to *"the default setting is that the records belong to the provider who has the control over it."* This is in contrast to doctors who, although they are required to store and protect health records, often believe it is the patient who ultimately owns them. *"My understanding is that patients have a legal right to their medical records when they request them. The physician is the caretaker and has the responsibility for maintaining those medical records."*[47] The situation is much clearer for mental health records as the HIPAA states that these can be only be shared with other providers with the patient's permission.

If that was not complicated enough once data has been aggregated and de-identified the game changes. At this point it can be sold without patient permission. Indeed, the default for many EHR vendors has been that the physician gives them the right to commercialize, de-identified and aggregated data. Currently individuals have no way of tracking this. While HIPPA privacy regulation gives patients the right to review and inspect their personal records, sometimes for a fee, tracing how they are being used once de-identified is pretty much impossible.

CUSTODIANSHIP

Some argue that the current regulation has made the assumption that health organisations should host and therefore control individuals' data. The consequence of this is that in several circumstances patient needs have become secondary to those of the healthcare system. This is why some, especially in Brussels, suggested that the debate should really focus on 'custodianship' identifying who is entrusted with guarding or maintaining health information and how they can be held to account for their actions. This can be considered from a number of different perspectives. For instance, in Western Australia and New South Wales, the Department of Health has a data stewardship policy which puts the focus on custodians managing data on behalf of the state not the patient.[48,49] In Canada, custodians are considered to be individuals or organisations that collect, maintain or use personal health information to provide or assist in the provision of health care or treatment.[50] Here they again have the interest of their employer at the fore but are obliged to respect the wishes of individuals to access or correct their records. Scotland's regional health polices include guidance on providing data to researchers, taking into account the public interest vs individual patient privacy.[51]

TRANSPARENCY

In other countries the situation is no less complicated. But, as understanding grows, so too does concern about how to control data access. To address this one approach is to be more transparent. An early mover here can be found in Denmark where, since 2003, sunhed.dk, an internet-based portal, provides access to medical records for both citizens and health care professionals.[52] Although initially mainly used by GPs, public access has increased substantially in recent years. Some of the big corporates have also tried to improve transparency – but so far with limited success. Microsoft's HealthVault, which launched in 2007 is just one of several opt-in platforms which seeks to enable patients to gather, store, use and share health information.[53] Bringing together medical information from providers and personal data, it expanded from the US to the UK in 2010. Google's version of this, Google Health, closed down in 2012 due to lack of adoption.

Also in the US, one of the most significant initiatives has been Open Notes which now provides over 20m US patients with the ability to review their medical records and report any discrepancies online. In addition, it reminds patients of important next steps, such as diagnostic and screening tests, referrals, and immunizations. Initial evaluations have suggested that this movement may increase patient activation and engagement in important ways and has shown that users have gained greater understanding (of health information), built better relationships (with doctors), received better quality care (adherence and compliance) and improved self-care (patient-centeredness, empowerment).[54]

REGULATION

In Europe, as highlighted in the privacy and security chapter, GDPR regulations are designed to encourage organisations to give back control of personal data to the individual. Although not specific around ownership, these regulations make it easier for individuals to access data which is held on them and to be able to change the permissions they grant for it to be used or shared. The UK is building on this approach and the NHS now states, *"every citizen will be able to access their full health records at the click of a button, detailing every visit to the GP and hospital, every prescription, test results, and adverse reactions and allergies."*[55] It is clear that, despite its rocky start, the push for transparency marks a significant step towards giving patients more control, and possibly ownership, of their personal information.

It is however India that currently stands out as one of the few nations where the issue is clearly defined. Here the National Health Portal has for some time had guidelines for patient data[56] which state that the *"physical or electronic records, which are generated by the healthcare provider, are held in trust by them on behalf of the patient,"* but that *"the contained data in the record which are the protected health information of the patient is owned by the patient himself / herself."* Patients can not only inspect the information, but also *"have the privileges to restrict access to and disclosure of individually identifiable health information."*

GREATER CONTROL

Whatever the approach, across all our discussions the assumption was that in the future patients will have greater control of their data and be able to access to more information. However, the interpretation of 'control' is varied. Key questions which have yet to be answered concern the benefits of full versus partial control, the link between control and responsibility as well as the improved use of data to give patients a better understanding of their health care choices. In some locations, the debate was around what really constitutes legal ownership – with insurance, pharmaceutical and care provider sectors all suggesting that individuals would not benefit from having sole control of their health data. Others consider that the issue is more about the ability for individuals and organisation to access and use data. *"Patients will have ability to opt-in and opt-out of data sharing and also correct errors."* In other words, it is really all about access vs. ownership?

INDIVIDUAL OVERSIGHT

It is within this area that platforms like **digi.me** (see case study) are now increasingly active. Starting with a pilot in Iceland and now moving to Norway, Australia and the UK, this is enabling citizens to download a copy of all their health data. At its core the aim is to deliver the ambition for individual oversight of all their health data, whatever the source and so put the patient 'in control' of how this is used. In addition, with organisations such as **Nebula Genomics** (see case study) giving the patient the ownership and control of their DNA profiles, the ability for individuals to further control and monetize their health data is moving forward.

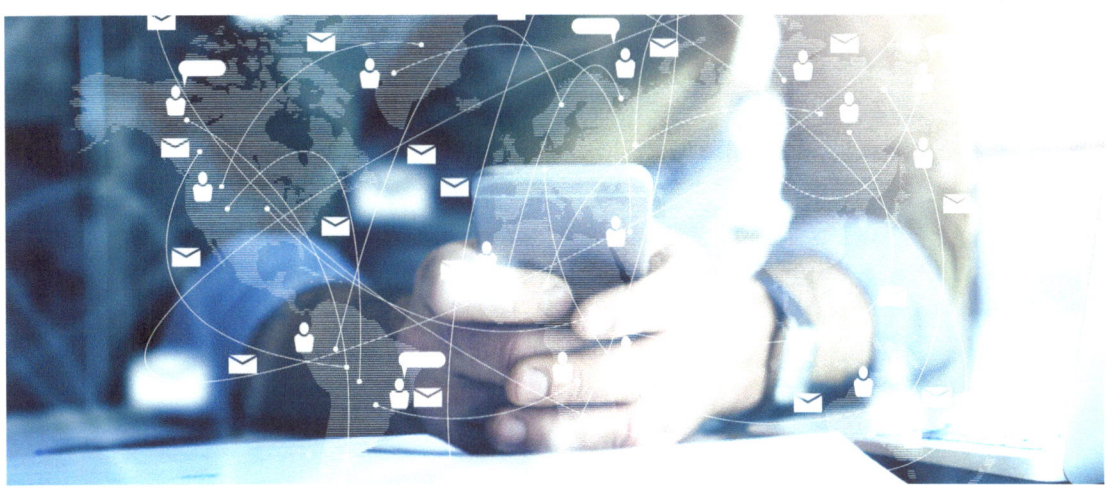

In our London discussion, several highlighted the UK Databox research project[57] which focuses on enhancing accountability and giving individuals control over the use of their personal data. This envisions *"an open-source personal networked device or service, that collates, curates, and mediates access to an individual's personal data by verified and audited third party applications and services. It will form the heart of an individual's personal data processing ecosystem, providing a platform for managing secure access to data and enabling authorised third parties to provide the owner with authenticated services, including services that may be accessed while roaming outside the home environment."*

Several organisations who 'can own the patient throughout the whole journey' are confident in their ability to manage access to information through 'joined-up health services' but without having to share data with other companies. Indeed, some felt that *"in 10 years, we will have solved the ambiguity of who owns what."* As *"decision making moves from experts to expert systems"* then maybe the data just becomes an input, or it is transparently monetized and used by all? This may be particularly relevant as *"insurers increasingly need the patient to be part of the system and hit targets (e.g. BMI measures)."* Although some questioned *"if fear of data overload will exceed the individuals' capacity to see things in perspective,"* others put the future focus very much on the capability of healthcare systems as a whole to *"give choice to individual"* and so enable the *"ability to see and correct your own data."*

Although varied jurisdictions may adopt different approaches and there may be no universal answer, a good number of organisations are already laying the ground for a world in which control of personal data does indeed shift (back) to the individual. The appetite is certainly evident. In Singapore, the view is that *"we will see more democratisation of health information and that is a good thing,"* while in Norway it was proposed that *"patients will become more health literate and so increasingly empowered,"* and hence this will *"drive individual responsibility and accountability that will deliver positive change."*

Benefits for the Patient

Foremost, giving greater visibility on all the health information that exists about an individual is itself a major advance on today. Linking in the ability to then question it and also control it in terms of granting permissions for access to trusted parties takes patient data an important further step forward. While not all may engage, for those that want to, then this shift to custodianship of one's personal data – from across all sources – holds the key for wider empowerment in the years ahead.

CASE STUDY:

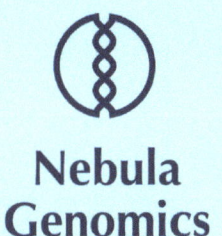

Companies such as 23andMe and AncestryDNA charge consumers under $200 to learn about their health or origins; others undertake whole genome sequencing for around $1,000. But all these companies retain control of the data: The customers / patients have no ownership. Co-founded by Harvard DNA sequencing pioneer George Church, MIT start-up Nebula Genomics is seeking to upend this 'exploitation'. It will offer whole genome sequencing, but allow customers to keep custodianship of their data, which they can then rent to the drug companies they choose, potentially making a profit in the process.[58]

Pharma and biotech companies spend billions of dollars each year to acquire genomic data and scientists need large genomic datasets to identify causes of disease and develop cures. However, to date, growth of the genomic data market has been hindered by small data quantities, data fragmentation, lack of data standardization and slow data acquisition. Launched in Feb 2018, Nebula Genomics is leveraging block-chain to eliminate middlemen and empower people to own their personal genomic data. This will effectively lower sequencing costs and enhance data privacy, resulting in growth of genomic data.[59] The company is planning to "spur genomic data growth by significantly reducing the costs of personal genome sequencing, enhancing genomic data protection, enabling buyers to efficiently acquire genomic data, and addressing the challenges of genomic big data. We will accomplish this through decentralization, cryptography, and utilization of the block-chain."[60]

While there are other platforms where people can sell their genetic information online, none offer genome sequencing. Nebula's goal is to get the price of sequencing below $1,000 by working with biotech and pharma companies, which will subsidize a large share of the cost. In addition, people will be able to earn cryptocurrency in exchange for letting pharma companies use their data.[61] People who want to get their genomes sequenced through Nebula will pay with tokens, which will also be used by researchers and companies wanting to acquire that data. Initial modelling proposes that an individual could earn up to 50 times the cost of sequencing their genome – taking into account both what could be made from a lifetime of renting out their genetic data, and reductions in medical bills if the results throw up a potentially preventable disease.

As co-founder and former Google employee Kamal Obbad views it, "under the current system, personal genomics companies effectively own your personal genomics data, and you don't see any benefit at all."[62] Some see the real problem will be whether it is possible to keep the DNA data private while still allowing data buyers to compute on it. With Nebula's model the sequence would belong to the individual, so they could rent it out over and over, including to multiple companies simultaneously. The data buyer would never take ownership or possession of it – rather, it is stored by the individual with Nebula then providing a secure computation platform on which the data buyer could compute on the data. "You stay in control of your data and you can share it securely with who you want to."

CASE STUDY:

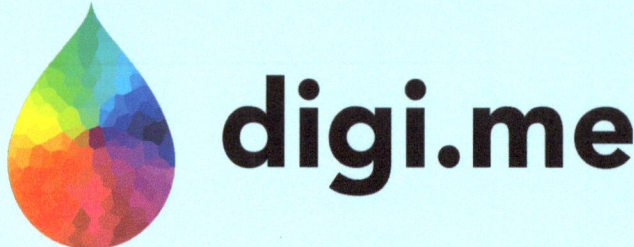

UK based digi.me is one of the leading personal data platforms. Operating across a number of sectors including both financial services and healthcare, it allows individuals to connect together multiple data sources.[63] From social media feeds and banking to wearables and health records, it enables users to have a secure personal data library on one of several major cloud-based platforms such as DropBox and Google Drive.

At its core the aim is to deliver the ambition for individual oversight of all their health data, whatever the source and so put the patient 'in control' of how this is used. Linking into personalised healthcare services and treatment its major 2017 pilot has been in Iceland where, as a world-first living lab project, all citizens have universal access to their healthcare data.[64] Iceland is now building on this base to create a broader personal data ecosystem. Other nations are expected to follow suit.

With the advent of GDPR across Europe and US regulation requiring healthcare providers to all create citizen-facing APIs to enable automated data download, the company is expanding quickly. Having merged with its US rival personal.com, digi.me is now working in partnership with a number of EU health systems as well as over 100 healthcare providers in the US via formats including Epic, Cerner and Blue Button. As the global ambition for more patient control of their data, many see digi.me and similar platforms setting the standards.

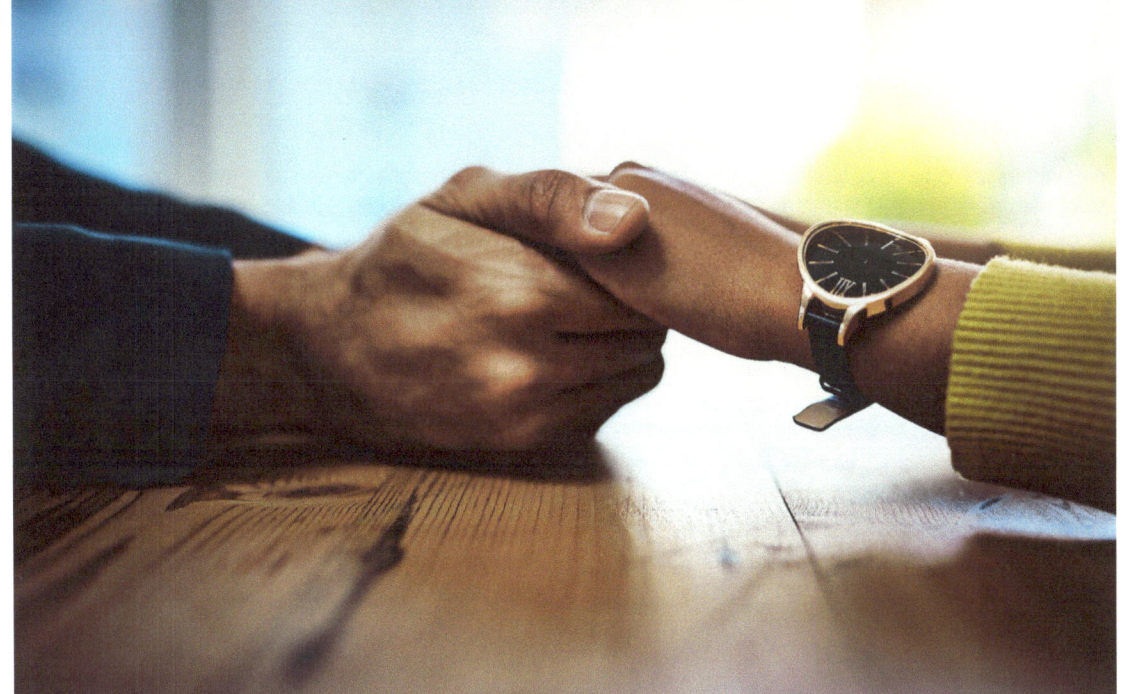

Trust

In many regions, trust needs to be (re)built between payers, providers and patients as well as with new entrants coming into the healthcare arena. New technology platforms and improving communication with the public both play a major role. Concern about ulterior motives for the use of data is high and some see AI adding to the challenge. Many recognise the need for greater transparency on practice in some pivotal areas.

Trust has traditionally been considered a cornerstone of effective doctor – patient relationships. The need for interpersonal trust relates to the vulnerability associated with being ill, the information asymmetries arising from the specialist nature of medical knowledge, and the uncertainty regarding the competence and intentions of the practitioner on whom the patient is dependent. Without trust patients may well not access services at all, let alone disclose all medically relevant information. Trust is also important at an institutional level, as trust in particular hospitals, insurers and health care systems may affect patient support for and use of services and thus their economic and political viability. Furthermore, without trust it would be almost impossible to carry out effective clinical trials and health research. Another fundamental problem with today's system is that patients lack knowledge and control.

In what has come to be called the post-traditional order the balance of trust is shifting. The days of 'doctor knows best', when patients blindly trusted in and deferred to medical expertise, are being challenged. At the same time breaches in patient data have undermined trust still more. A 2017 survey from Accenture revealed that cyber-attacks have already affected more than one in every four people in the US resulting in an average of $2,500 out-of-pocket costs. Technology has opened the door to vast sources of information and, with various degrees of accuracy, consumers can often self-diagnose, their condition with few choice words and a google search. Today the consumer is 'king' and the 'informed patient' frequently expects to play an active part in decision-making regarding their treatment.[65]

TRUSTED SOURCES

Access to trusted sources of information is therefore essential in supporting consumers as they consider treatment options, shop for health care, and select, buy, and use their health insurance. Yet it seems that many of the trusted sources fall outside the traditional health care system, demonstrating that not just the information but also the information source matters. Looking beyond the immediate patent doctor relationship we are now in a world where, with exception of maybe Canada, the Nordics and Singapore, many regions, public trust in established institutions, especially government, is in deterioration. In South Africa, trust in the national government and the private sector is, for example, pretty low. In several locations we visited, the focus was on how little trust there is between different services – social care, health, aging services etc. and how to use data to build bridges between the different silos.

TRANSPARENCY

We are evidently in a state of flux as, for some, trust has moved away from institutions such as government and the established brands to centre on personal networks. This is having a significant impact on health care delivery. As Eric Topol shared powerfully in his influential 2015 book *'The Patient Will See You Now'* we are entering *"a new era in trust and transparency."*

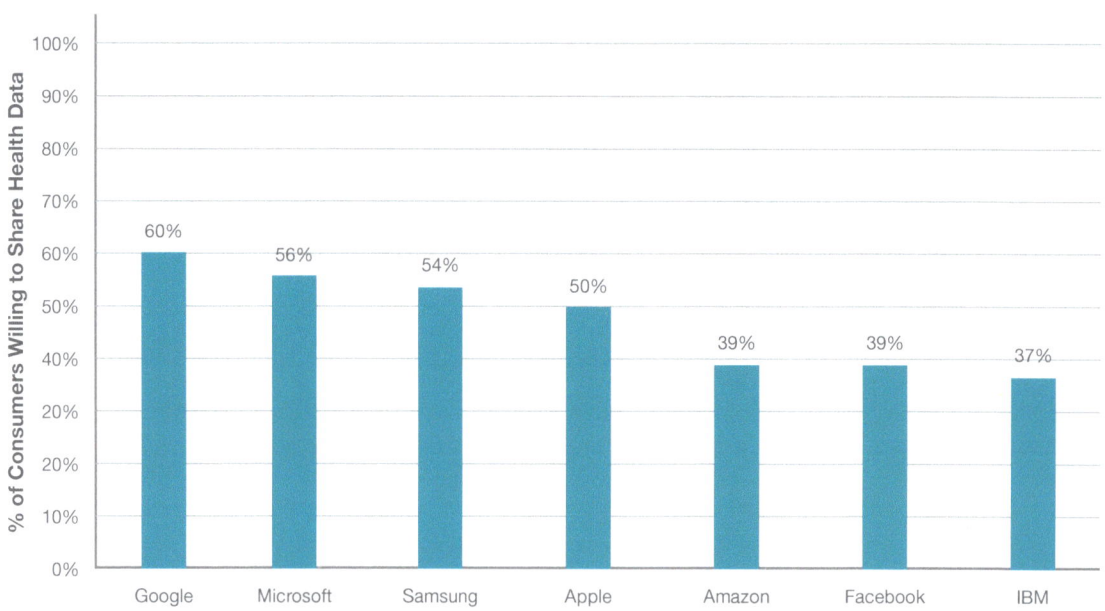

Consumers Willing To Share Health Data

Source: Rock Health 2016 Consumer Survey

The Edelman trust barometer has for several years highlighted that healthcare as a sector is near the bottom of the rankings alongside financial services. In particular, as trust in pharmaceutical companies continues to slide, *"lesser trust in pharma and biotech companies carries with it broad implications for the ability to attract and keep employees, license to operate in the larger health and business ecosystem, and greater support for regulations that may threaten a license to lead."*[66] Less than half the population trusts healthcare company CEOs and only 70% of employees who work in the healthcare sector say they trust the company for which they work. For healthcare generally, the largest gaps in consumer expectations and how they see healthcare performing lie in the areas of transparency.

As shown in the chart below, very recently there has been good levels of trust in big tech. In 2016, over half of the Americans surveyed in one study said that they were willing to share health data with Google, Microsoft, Samsung or Apple. However, with growing anxiety over such issues as privacy, taxation and fake news, confidence in much of the big tech sector is also falling – just as many are seeking to move deeper into the health sector. This is a big concern for healthcare as many of the new partnerships around better use of patient data are built around collaboration with some of the companies in the spotlight. So, what can be done to address this?

BUILDING TRUST

Implicit within many discussions on how the future of patient data may evolve is the issue of building greater trust. This is not just in terms of personal trust between the patient and the multiple public-facing elements within the health care system, but also regarding the growing cohort of hidden partners that manage, store and utilise patient information. Many agree that *"if patients are to willingly share their data, and if multiple organisations are going to collaborate, there has to be a higher level of public trust than currently exists."*

In Sydney, it was agreed that good regulation is key: *"from a policy perspective, we need to be clear who owns what data and who can share what. We also need to know what information can be accessed in an emergency vs. what data will always requires consent from the individual. This will enable us to agree the right standards and set clear roles."* Broader views on where greater transparency may help to build trust include the pricing and efficacy of drugs. Particular examples highlighted the better use of taxation and how to link funding levels to outcome measures for interventions.

Many believe that one of the most effective ways to build trust is by making information more accessible. *"We need a digital transformation that makes everything easy to use with market and social forces aligning so we can move to better health outcomes based on personalized data."* Many again mentioned Iceland as leading in this space. There citizens are given access to digital copies of all their health data. In London, it was suggested that better communication would do much to build public trust: *"We have to address culture as a barrier to change"* and *"we need to differentiate between real risks and the myths (that are often driven by the media). Key is creating more positive storytelling."* Significantly, *"we need positive early stories to share alongside experiences that matter. There should be clear mutual propositions for sharing and improving transparency."* Beyond this there was agreement that patients should be given greater advice and support so that they can more easily decide what is advisable to share and be given clear choices around whether they should do so – especially on sensitive issues such as sexual or mental health.

BLOCK-CHAIN

Given that one way to establish trust is to increase transparency, several expect that block-chain will have a role to play. The view in South Africa for example was that, despite its limitations, *"we are confident in the security provided by block-chain in terms of it being more difficult to hack but we recognize that it is not as efficient as other options."*

The Canadian government is also investigating block-chain's potential and participants in the Toronto workshop proposed that *"smart contracts may be the best way to utilize it: When more data is liberated then block-chain may have a greater role to play."* But this *"will not impact healthcare 'at scale' in the next 10 years."* Others see that *"using block-chain for health records is a possibility but the idea that this can backdate and work on legacy systems is stretching it too far."* Some consider it to be just more hype and suggest that the noise around this new technology might damage the health debate. *"If we believe trust is an incomplete contract then block-chain is a useful technical tool but doesn't solve the fundamental issue. There are many false expectations and naïve views of block-chain."*

Block-chain has captured the imagination of the healthcare industry, from payers and providers, through pharmacies and product providers. The peer-to-peer network that replaces the traditional role of a centrally trusted authority. More are seeing that leveraging block-chain as a shared bundled-payment platform between providers and payers, greater transparency of price, cost and quality data could be achieved, helping to alleviate the mistrust. In recent Cognizant research, how organisations are planning to use block-chain within healthcare was however notably varied. 44% are planning to adopt a permissioned block-chain that is only accessible to trusted participants while 38% said they are planning to adopt a public block-chain.[67]

Several companies are being proactive about how to use block-chain as part of the mix. Nebula Genomics for one is making interesting moves around allowing patients to own and monetize their DNA profiles. Emin Gün Sirer, co-director of the Initiative for Cryptocurrencies and Smart Contracts at Cornell University has commented that *"the idea of trying to get individuals to monetise their own genomes using the block-chain is an interesting and new one."*[68]

MANAGING DISTRUST

Many are increasingly wary about some of the motivations behind the collection of data. The question raised in Dubai was *"to what extent can we trust organisations who collect and manage our more personalized data and, in particular, our DNA / genomic profiles?"* And then *"how will employers or government use the new health data? Will they select and prioritize treatment and coverage? Is that the natural next stage of health insurance?"* Moreover, "if employers can identify (and recruit) the best and healthiest then what will happen to everyone else? What will happen to those with mental health issues? If the information is available to them, will employers refuse to recruit people who may be prone to depression?" Finally, some ask *"what role can the government play to help manage the problem?"*

In a bespoke workshop with a UK health insurance company, this issue was seen as a major business risk – especially if it raises public concerns which are then fanned by gossip and media speculation. This really is an important issue. As more accurate health data is generated, the possibility that it could be accessed and misused will be impossible to ignore. *"Insurance companies cannot mandate genetic tests, but they may need to differentiate between customers who have them and those who do not."*

In Sydney, the view was that *"no one wants to see a future where genetic profiling means that individuals are excluded from healthcare cover and wider economic or social engagement, such as employment. However, it could happen."* One suggested response was maybe *"insurance companies need to steer clear of using genetic data in any significant way in order to ensure that customers do not feel that they could be penalized."* Traditional risk analysis based on family history and blood tests etc., may well remain the standard point of reference for premium calculation - even though more detailed information is clearly going to be available.

Back in London, this point unpacked wider concerns about the business model for health insurance. Comments included; *"insurance needs to stop looking at data and start sharing"* and *"putting people into smaller and smaller boxes is hugely unhelpful. Some risks are not diversifiable if you shrink the pool so that it becomes impractical."* Several see that the model for health insurance is currently very primitive and if it is to have relevance in the future then how patient data is used and managed will be critical: *"We assume we are giving our data to someone we trust but organisations (such as Experian for instance) are already gathering it and selling it back to other companies."* With more and better personal information increasingly available over the next decade then a huge 'tsunami of change' may be heading the way of the insurance sector.

THE ROLE OF AI

Many are also concerned about the challenges that AI will uncover – particularly as vulnerable patients might find themselves exploited by increasingly intelligent algorithms. Some are already more comfortable communicating sensitive health issues to electronic devices, machines and chat-bots, rather than humans. What happens if they begin to be manipulated by them? What would happen if an algorithm taught itself a new way to question health data? In the same way that Google Translate AI invented its own language,[69] we risk losing control of our ability to interrogate health data and AI decision-making. The perceptions of trust in how the privacy of NHS patients was treated in the early stages of the partnership with Deep Mind was mentioned several times.[70]

HUMAN TOUCH

Alongside all the technological developments in the mix including wider block-chain use, one company specifically highlighted in Sydney is taking a more human approach to increasing trust in its field of focus. One of the top insights from the 2015 Future Agenda programme was that *"as service provision and consumption becomes ever more digital, automated and algorithmic, those brands that can offer more emotional engagement and human-to-human contact become increasingly attractive."*[71]

In a world of more automation in healthcare, **Flatiron** (see case study) is using a team of humans to sort through patient records and identify the critical data points. Technology cannot yet deal with the unstructured information within which exist the vital signals that point to specific cancer diagnosis, and so the company is using *"human-mediated extraction of data describing human illness, to achieve a level of utility required and explicitly demanded by the human physicians caring for patients, by the human researchers developing new medicines, and by the human regulators evaluating their efforts."*[72] Flatiron has built trust with a very particular community of oncologists and has done it so well that Roche has recently acquired it for over $2bn.

Benefits for the Patient

Without trust in the system and healthcare organisations, patients will not be willing to share the all-important data. Whether through better technology or more human touch in the critical moments of truth, building more trust is a primary motivation for many across the sector. Getting this right at a time when trust itself is in such flux is not going to be easy, but it is going to be essential.

CASE STUDY:

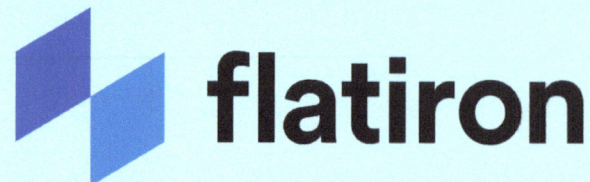

An Alphabet-backed start-up, Flatiron has a very different approach to Google. Rather than selling access to users, it provides access to de-identified, aggregated clinical information with a particular focus on cancer. Success is driven by understanding what practicing oncologists really see as meaningful and providing clear value that can help in treating patients. Core to achieving this is a dataset that is distinct in the industry. Flatiron has a "meticulously assembled oncology dataset that pulls information from the electronic health records and organizes it in a fashion that approaches the quality of clinical research, enabling investigators (and regulators) to ask questions of the data that might normally require a dedicated, stand-alone study to resolve."[73]

Given that so much of the available, real-world clinical data is unstructured and stored across thousands of disconnected community clinics, medical centres and hospitals, the core challenge is making sense of all this information. 'In cancer, many of the critical data points reside in documents that are not structured at all. For example, histology. If a cancer is an adenocarcinoma or a squamous cell cancer is something that's in a pathology report, and sometimes it's really distinct, and it's pretty easy to pull that information out. But a lot of the times, it's contextual, and includes a lot of the other information that a pathologist is seeing. And this is not just histology, but information like biomarkers, and what's in the radiology report, and what's in the clinical case notes. 50% or more the critical data points you need for research live in these PDF representations of data."[74]

The company sees that "each patient's story has the unique potential to teach us something new about the way cancer works, and help us find more effective treatments, faster."[75] As such, and given its' heritage, it is notable in its' very human approach. Working with 2m active patients' records, at its core are a sizable team of healthcare professionals who are reading through the unstructured data to extract key insights. While 'technology-enabled' with underlying systems to monitor accuracy and match

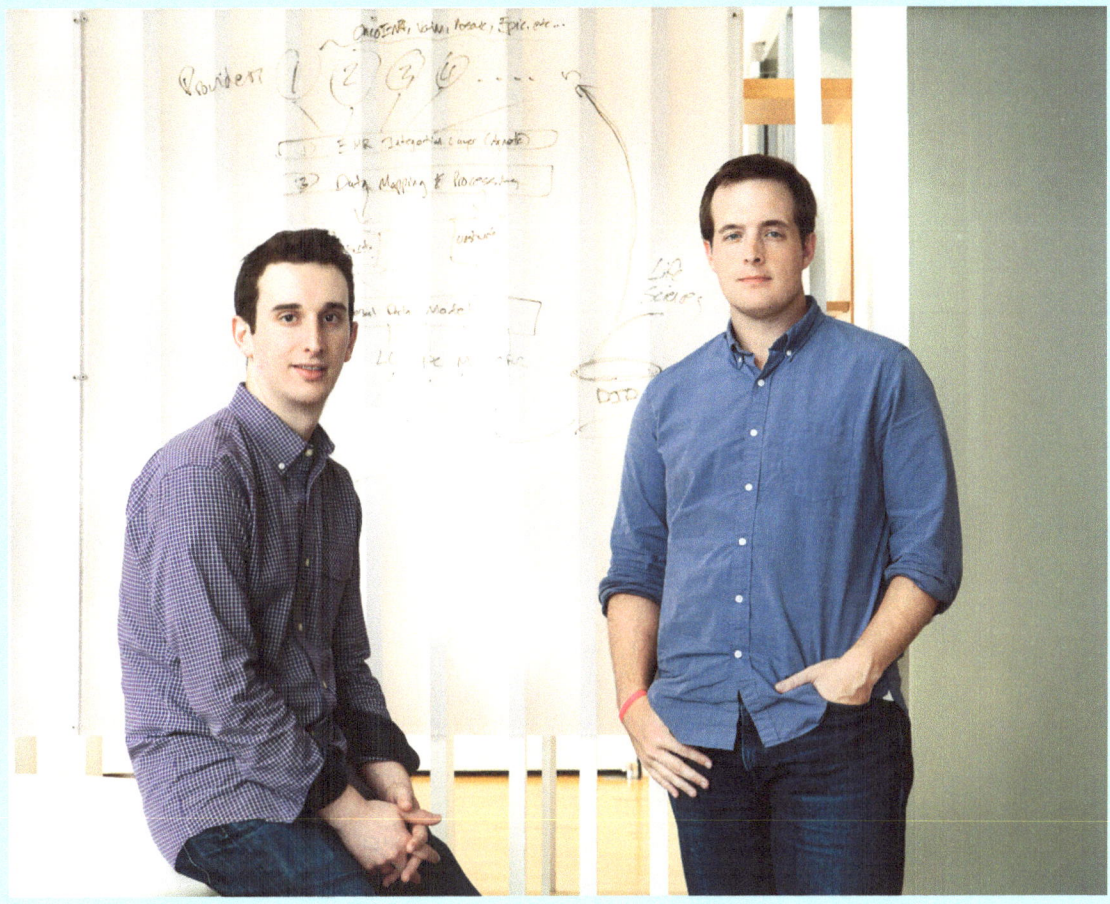

information to structured data, the essential work is being done by human beings. Going forward, some expect that AI may deliver efficiency benefits but, for now, the key capability is "human-mediated extraction of data describing human illness, to achieve a level of utility required and explicitly demanded by the human physicians caring for patients, by the human researchers developing new medicines, and by the human regulators evaluating their efforts."[76]

In 2018, Flatiron was acquired by pharma company Roche for a not-insignificant $2.1bn – many expect it to provide access to real world data from a network of oncology practices that can be used to provide a trusted, clinical-research grade record of drug efficacy and utility. This offers the possibility of obtaining regulator-worthy data with unprecedented ease, saving significant money from clinical study costs and delivering the relevant data for quicker decisions - and a faster time-to-market. Flatiron has achieved a level of physician-engineer collaboration that most health tech companies fail to approach and has also strategically partnered closely with regulators, providing FDA with complimentary access to data, and publishing together the results of such analyses. "This helped the company refine the platform, better understanding the questions they should be addressing, while also providing referenceability for pharma companies: if Flatiron data is good enough to be used by the FDA, it's worthy of pharma attention as well."[77] Now with the support of Roche, Flatiron Health is building its capacity to turn health data into insights – "transforming EHR data into analysable, actionable information."

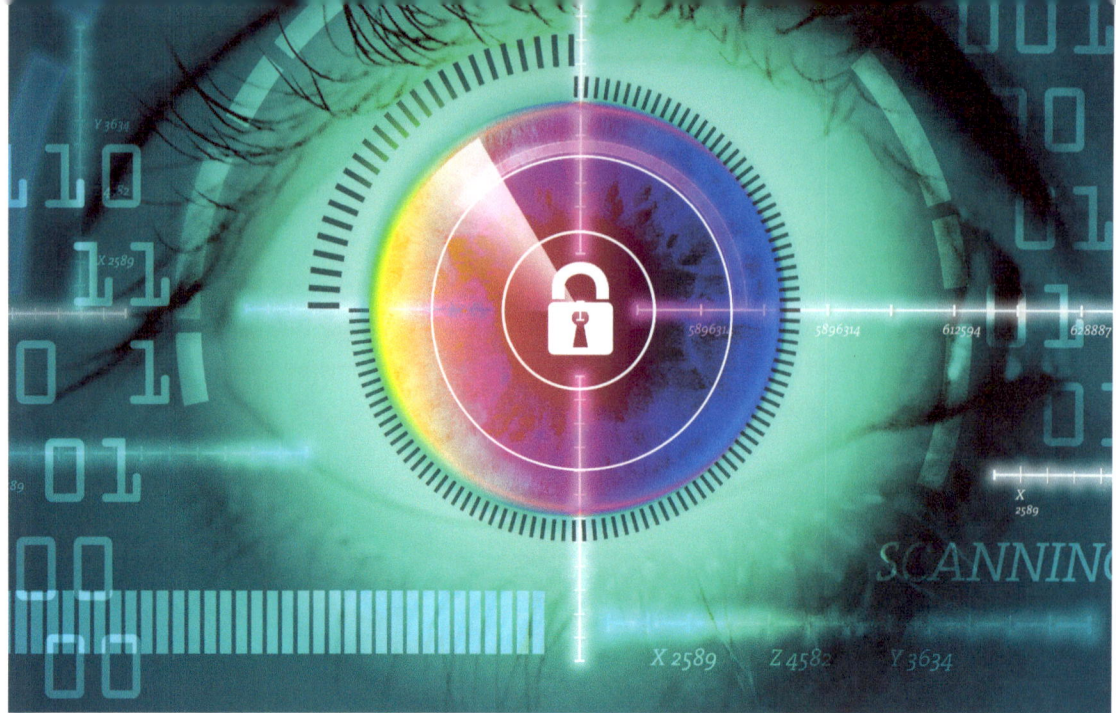

Security and privacy

As anonymized, aggregated data is more easily re-linked and sensitive health data is a target for cyber-attacks, questions are raised around the benefits of centralized vs. decentralized data and the impact of localization. Given both the sensitivity and value of healthcare data it is little surprise that security and privacy are high on multiple agendas. As vulnerability and risk increase apace with greater focus from external hackers and internal sources, these are growing concerns for many.

Throughout previous Future Agenda discussions on the future of data and privacy, the vulnerability of health data to hacking has been consistently highlighted. Back in 2010 at a lunch in Washington DC, a prediction was made that *"in the future there will be a 'privacy Chernobyl' that will fundamentally change our attitudes to sharing information."* When pushed to highlight how this may happen, the expert view then was that it would most likely be in US health data as the information has high value, relatively low security (compared to passports and financial services) and lacks agreed standards. Eight years later, a view in San Francisco was that *"Equifax[78] is the canary in the coalmine – and healthcare information is way more valuable than financial information. It is up to 200 x more valuable (especially in a fragmented healthcare system where fraud is possible)."* Today almost a quarter of all data breaches in America happen in health care. In 2015, over 113m Americans' healthcare records were compromised.

THE SECURITY CHALLENGE

Medical data is indeed a popular target for criminals. As highlighted in the graph from FT research below, the average cost per capita of a health data breach in 2017 was calculated to be $380, way more than the $240 for financial data and significantly greater than any other sector. Reuters estimates that medical information is worth 10 times more than credit card information on the black market. Healthcare data can be monetised.

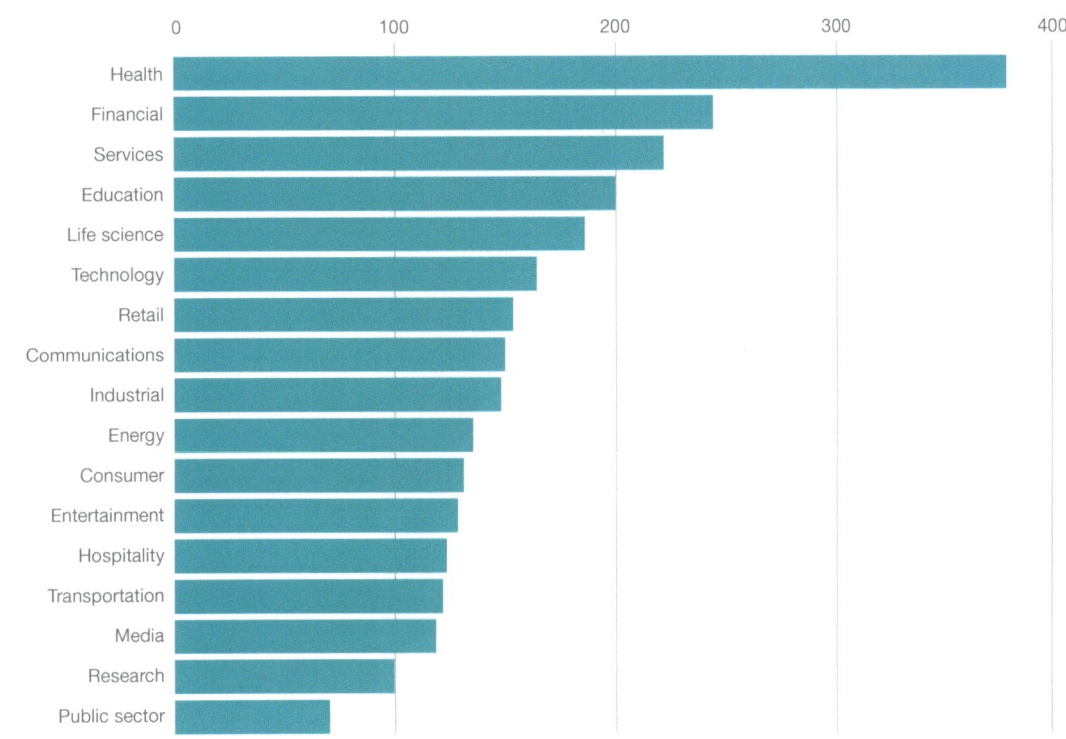

Data Breach Cost Per Capita

By industry classification, 2017 ($)

Source: Ponemon Institute / FT

The latest analysis of the world's biggest data breaches (see chart) reveals not only the growing number of attacks but also some of the most significant.[79] Although the 3bn user information Yahoo hack of 2013 is still the largest data hack to date in terms of absolute numbers of accounts compromised, many point to the 2015 breach that gained data on 78.8m customers of Anthem, the second-largest health insurer in the U.S, as having greater financial value.[80] Records accessed included names, dates of birth, social security numbers, addresses, emails and phone numbers. Similar information was gleaned from 4.5m records at Community Health Systems in 2014 and 4m at Advocate Medical Group a year earlier. Although these are also minor in terms of numbers of users when compared to others, given the higher multiples evidently attached to health data, the potential total financial impact of the data loss is far greater.

World's Biggest Data Breaches

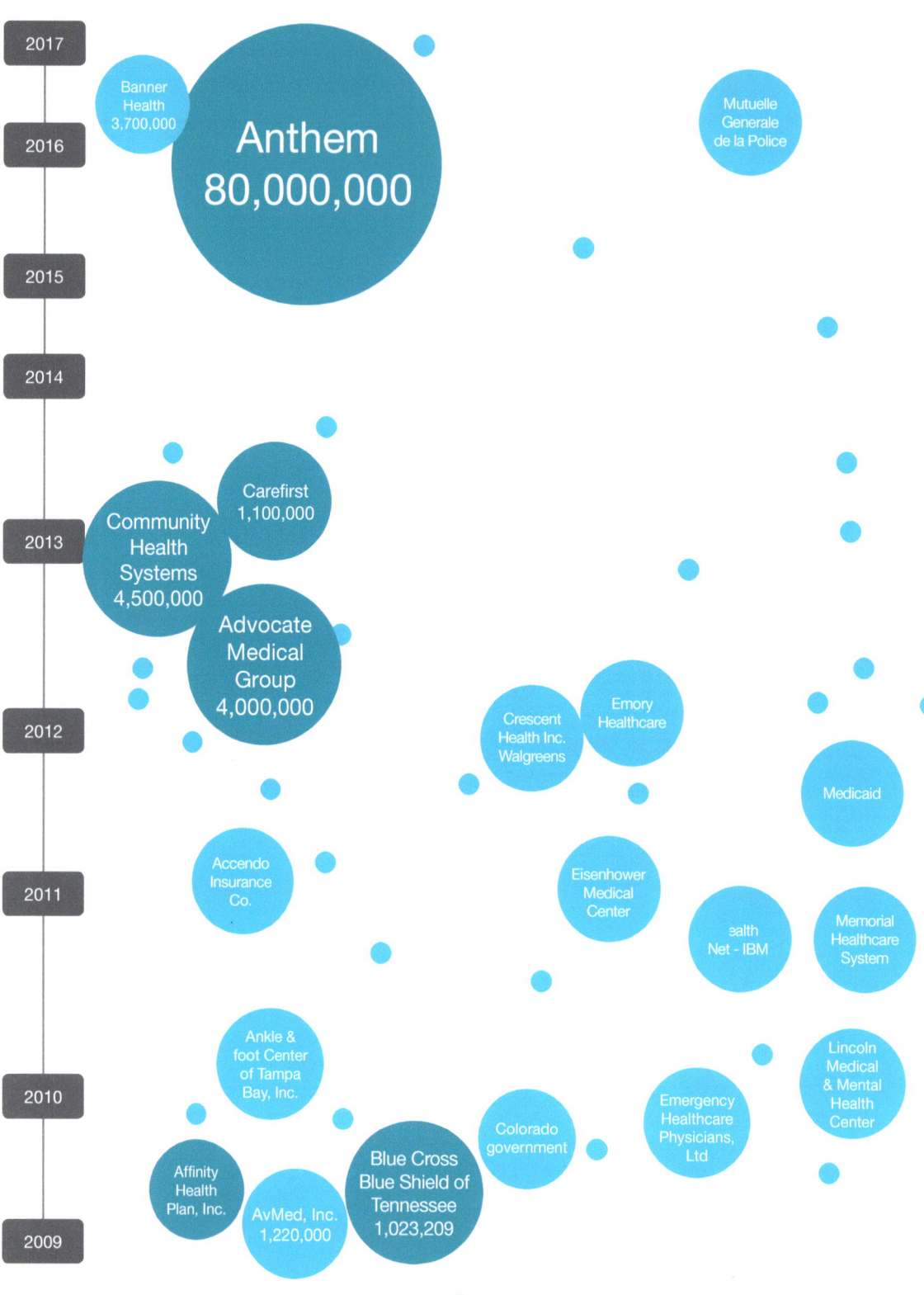

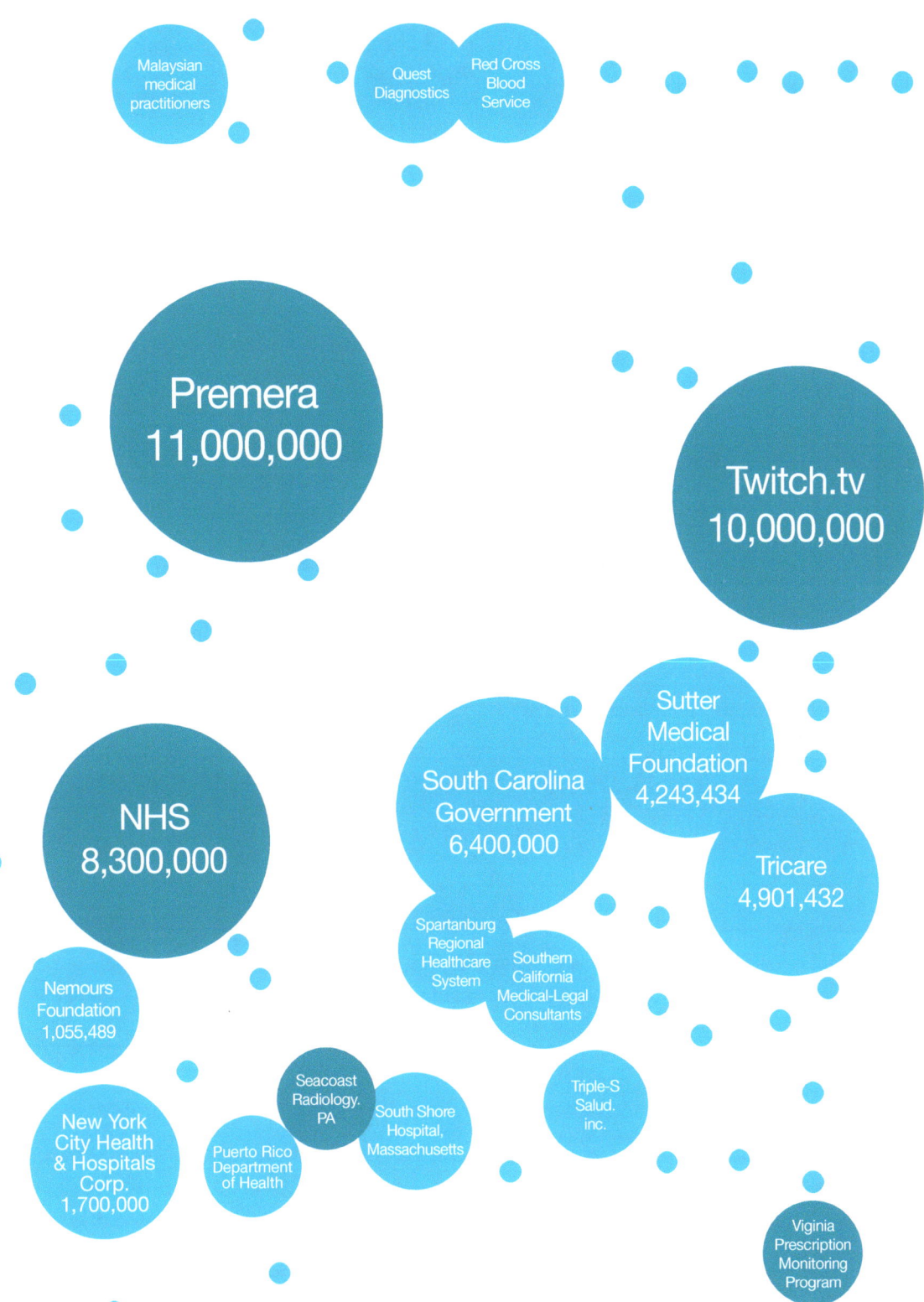

MALWARE

However, while these are significant in terms of value perhaps it was the 2017 infection of a third of the UK's NHS systems as part of the WannaCry malware attack that raised wider concerns on future disruption and data vulnerability.[81] This brought key parts of a national healthcare system to a halt, leading to over 600 cancelled operations and appointments and highlighted that few hospitals had the latest software updates. Ransomware presents an easier and safer way for hackers to gain cash; and, given the potential disruption, most organisations opt to simply pay the ransom. This has unintended consequences of funding more research by attackers who in turn develop more sophisticated and targeted attacks.[82] What is increasingly clear is that the more patient data is stored, shared and analysed in the cloud or shared with different firms, the greater the potential threat of hacking or misuse.

KPMG is just one of many organisations calling for improved security: *"Protecting patients' individual rights, including their personal data needs to be as important as the treatment they receive."* But was is to be done? Cisco, for instance, sees that as well as detecting and preventing malware, securing health and care communities in the future will also require greater cognizance of the vulnerability from the IoT and more connected homes, hospitals and care facilities.[83] Others see that maybe this is more than a traditional security risk.

CYBER-ATTACKS

Beyond financial gain, across all our discussions there was general acknowledgement that health data is increasingly vulnerable to a cyber-attack and there is a pressing need to address the problem. Some are even proposing that health firms should face stringent penalties if they are slapdash about security. The responses to this vary significantly. In Singapore, the view is that there is *"potential future vulnerability to as yet unknown risk from cyber-attacks, coercion or even biological warfare informed by health data and this is why data cannot be shared beyond national boundaries."* Discussions in London and the US noted "focus on bio-warfare and destabilization" and the example mentioned several times (including in follow-on discussions in Bangkok) was the alleged activity of the USAF in mapping Russian genes,[84,85] and the capacity to make weapons that only target one race.

Although many focus on the external threats, most attacks and data breaches in the US system don't come from outside hackers: *"The majority of all inappropriate accesses to EHRs comes from the inside. They involve nurses or doctors, billing specialists, or administrators who have legitimate reasons for having access to systems but who abuse that access for revenge, financial gain or just plain curiosity."* In the US in 2016 there were 450 breaches, affecting 27 million patient records. Of those, 120 incidents were outside hacks, while 200 came from insider actions.[86] Not surprisingly there are many organisations seeking to prevent this or detect it. Protenus is just one of several start-ups focused on tracking behaviours of healthcare workers within hospitals and their access to patient data.[87] It is aiming to improve how healthcare organisations monitor patient data use and does this by using AI analytics to search out anomalous behaviours in health systems. It is effectively automatically policing patient data access and reporting potential breaches.

In its most recent data-breach forecast, Experian predicted that the healthcare sector would be the most heavily targeted industry.[88] It anticipates that "mega breaches will move on from focusing on healthcare insurers to other aspects of healthcare, including hospital networks. These more distributed networks present a ripe target for attackers as it is often harder to maintain security measures as compared to more centralised organisations."

How to store data effectively is another tricky area. *"Patient data appears to be equally vulnerable whether in one centralized database or if it is distributed."* One participant mentioned that *"we *have 60,000 files on AWS so I am concerned about hacking and breach potential."* Although Amazon is one of the more secure cloud services providers, anxiety is there. Finding the right balance to improve security, reduce risk and yet enable the wider sharing of patient data that many desire is going to be a difficult task. Although there is a growing political view in some regions that expresses the right to data privacy and the right to data security the reality is that *"both are illusions: Security is impossible without increased monitoring – and so true privacy is also impossible."*

THE PRIVACY CHALLENGE

In terms of privacy specifically there are mounting challenges and increasingly visibility. Organisations such as the IAPP have been offering advice on the topic for several years.[89] Privacy is now increasingly part of the mainstream conversation and after the recent Facebook / Cambridge Analytica revelations public awareness is rising dramatically. Its implications on healthcare and patient data are also growing. In the UK the NHS and DeepMind came under criticism for the way that the anonymized data of 1.6m patients was shared in 2016.[90]

Around the world, multiple legislative acts are already in place or emerging.

- In the US, health care privacy and security are governed by the Health Insurance Portability and Accountability Act (HIPAA). This limits disclosure of patient data and mandates secure storage and transmission of electronic records. Anybody who violates HIPAA faces civil and criminal penalties. So, the law ensures that providers and health plans take steps to protect your health data and that you retain important rights over how it is used. Similar regulation is in place in a number of locations.

- In force from May 2018 in EU, the GDPR regulation aims primarily to give control back to citizens and residents over their personal data. It sets clear principles that apply to all use of patients' data and to all data controllers.[91]

- In India, the Ministry of Health (MoHFW) has supported a sector-specific law on privacy.[92] Necessitated by the fact that interoperable EHRs are a key component of Digital India, the Healthcare Data Privacy and Security Act will develop a comprehensive legal framework for protection of individual health data and its standardisation and identify the 'ownership' of that data through the establishment of a national e-health authority and health information exchanges.

As highlighted in our project summary map, general privacy regulation is now considered by lawyers to be strong is a wide range of countries including the US, Canada, Western Europe, Australia, Singapore and South Korea and 'robust' in China, Japan, Central Europe and Argentina.[93] Privacy protection specific to health data is now growing in strength in other locations including India, Brazil and much of SE Asia.

ENCRYPTION

Given this, a major challenge is how to balance the level of encryption to preserve privacy while ensuring relevant data is accessible to doctors and so the system is efficient. Today, de-identified data that you share is driving the most important advance in medicine: population-based data discoveries and tools to manage our health, wellness, and diseases.[94] *"There is an illusion of anonymization."* Most agree that the risk of sharing data should be not only recognised, but also made more public. No one is guaranteeing that aggregated or anonymized data can be 100% secure, or that individuals cannot be traced from it, and so, maybe, patients should be made more aware of this? Others agreed that going forward *"no data will be truly anonymous"* and we will see different levels of re-identification. *"Much current health data practice assumes that technology will not be able to be relinked to its source. This is not the case."*

POTENTIAL SOLUTIONS

Addressing the security and privacy challenges while enabling greater patient data access and sharing is plainly a highly problematic balancing act. One proposal is to push anonymization to a greater level – hence the support for the likes of block-chain. Estonia, for instance, is already using block-chain to protect its' citizens medical data. But, while seeming to improve security, this could actually make much medical data more difficult to use for research purposes. A counter-question raised in Oslo was *"as clinical studies data is made more open and put into the public domain, how can we be confident that all will abide by the agreed rules of use?"* In Boston, another view was that the risks from identification of data will be controlled as the *"increasing volume of data being generated makes identification more difficult."* Moreover, *"data is increasingly temporary (e.g. Snapchat) – so the premise of relinking is not true."* Technology will solve the problem so as such the link-ability of open data problem is a *"failed response to managing big data."*

While some of this may be true, others are calling for systemic action.[95] As many healthcare organisations have been slow to adopt practices that have worked for other industries, many do not, for example, use multi-factor authentication. It is standard in financial services but not in healthcare. Going forward healthcare providers should 'apply strong encryption to all patient data and limit who has permission to access medical charts.' An Experian recommendation is that *"healthcare organisations of all sizes and types need to ensure they have proper, up to date security measures in place, including contingency planning for how to respond to a ransomware attack and adequate employee training about the importance of security."*[96] Others point to more bio-metric security as has already being integrated into the Indian Aadhaar system. Whatever approaches are adopted it is clear that if the ambition of wider collection and sharing of patient data is to progress, then a broadening range of security and privacy issues clearly have to be proactively addressed.

Benefits for the Patient

Without security and privacy in the healthcare system, there will be little trust. Without trust patients will not use new platforms nor will they be willing to share more of their personal information with existing healthcare organisations. This is a universal barrier to progress. As individual's digital footprints become more visible, more valuable and more vulnerable to misuse, patients will increasingly expect guarantees from care providers..

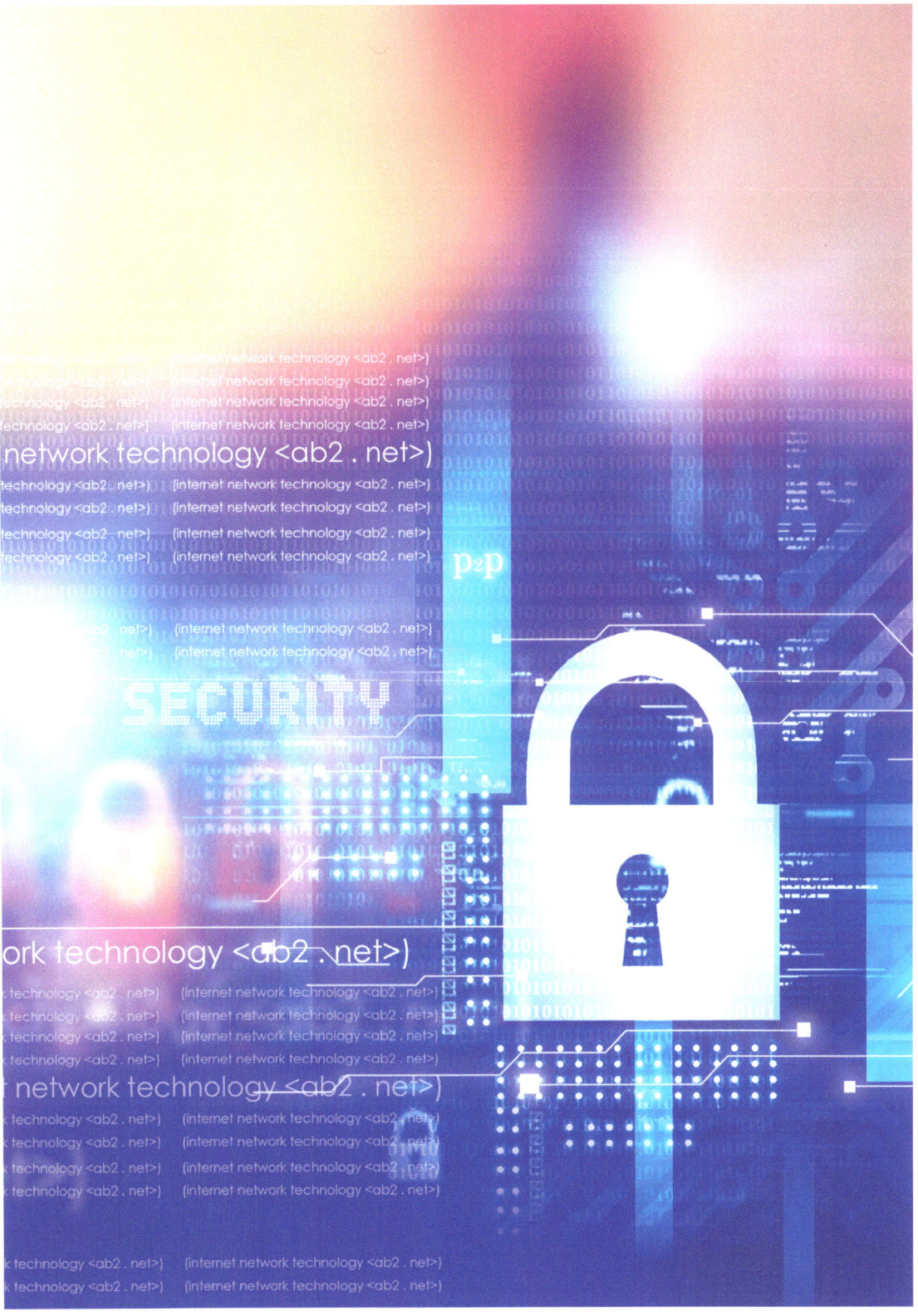

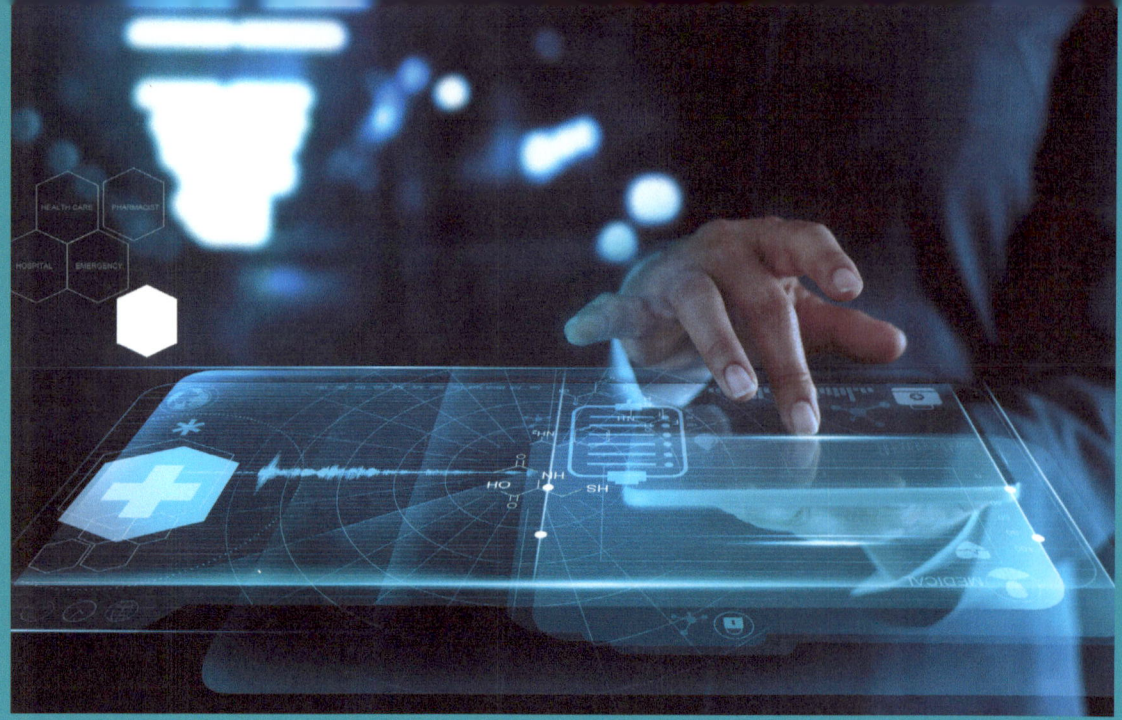

Future opportunities

Throughout our discussions there have been four key areas which are seen as major opportunities for patient data to improve efficiency and drive innovation. Although, again, not all are the same in the detail of execution in every location. This is often due to differing regulatory frameworks around privacy or the influence of a single payer system. However, they are all seen as major areas for potential change to occur over the next decade. Significant investment has already been made in some areas, both by government and the private sector. All are fields where there is tangible change to be delivered and, if undertaken in a coherent and effective manner, considerable benefits to be achieved.

These four areas are:

Personalisation – The prospect of more individualized 'n=1' healthcare is accelerating. Remote access, localised support and decision-making are all central to creating more personalized information which in turn will drive better healthcare. Predictive analytics and genetic profiling will further transform treatment: But will the benefits extend beyond the lucky few?

Data Marketplaces – Embedded in the future of access to patient data, is its wider exchange and what may be public commons vs. what is open for commercial purposes. Personal and clinical data will be represented in health data marketplaces that seek to both create financial value as well as enable better care. Given the value of health data in some key regions, marketplaces will undoubtedly expand but ensuring that the patient gains advantage will be pivotal.

The Impact of AI - There are great expectations around AI. Initial advances from machine learning and pattern recognition will be significant in enabling more efficient diagnosis and better prediction. As deep learning and self-learning then develop, the ability to deal with unstructured data delivers major improvements in diagnosis and treatment and AI is embedded into many clinical decisions. Moreover, with voice and facial recognition increasingly analysing users' behaviour patterns, AI is also applied to identify stress and anxiety.

New Models – While we will see some change from within, expect big tech, led especially by Amazon, to further disrupt health care. This will shift reimbursement mechanisms and drive shared risk across payers and providers. Equally significant change is emerging from China and India where the creation of identity related platforms is driving innovation at scale. At the same time, some anticipate that the reinvention of healthcare business models will come from more unexpected places.

Each of these are explored in the following pages.

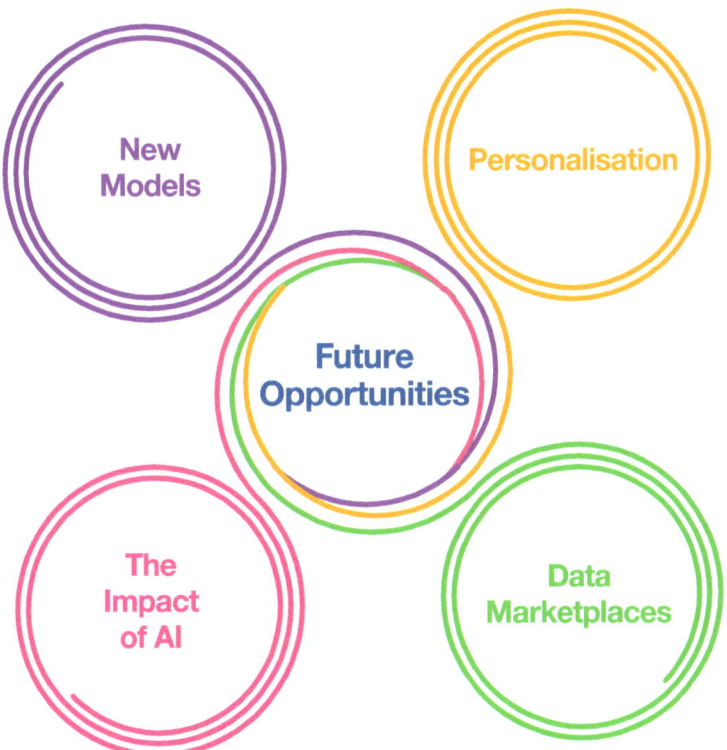

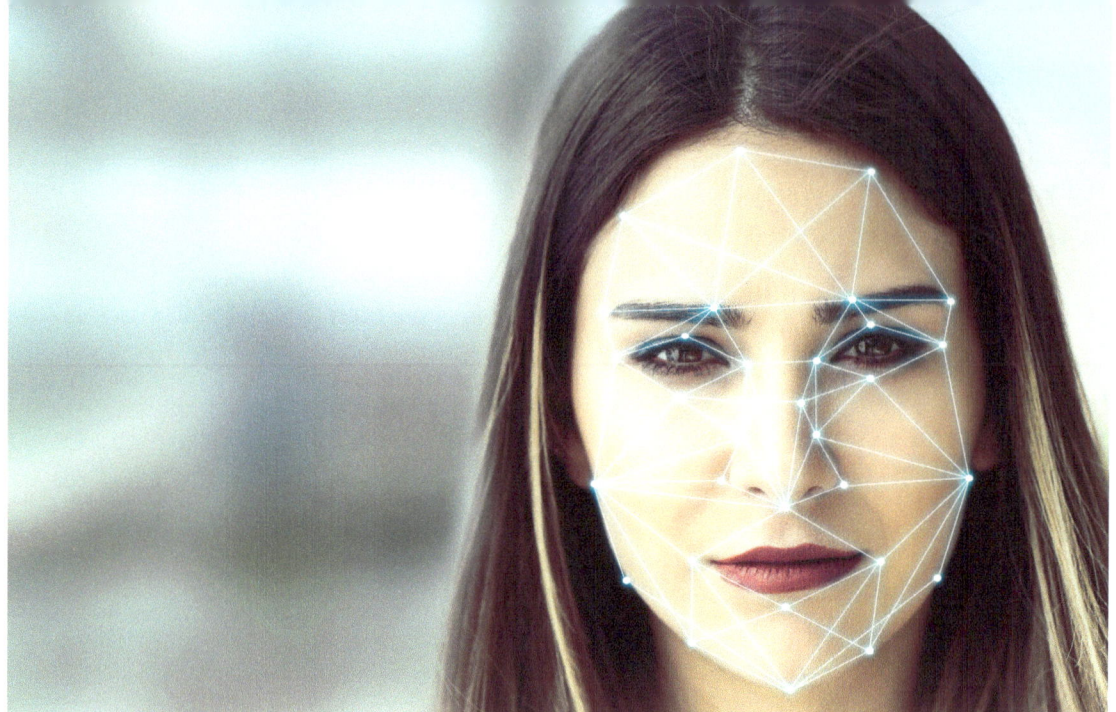

Personalisation

The prospect of more individualized 'n=1' healthcare is accelerating. Remote access, localised support and decision-making are all central to creating more personalized information that in turn will drive better healthcare. Predictive analytics and genetic profiling will further transform treatment: But will the benefits extend beyond the lucky few?

The consistent view in many locations we visited was that *"more detailed, personal information will help generate better health outcomes."* Therefore, better and more access to data about the individual is key to future healthcare delivery. This belief is driving much of the appetite for the collection, sharing and use of patient data.

GREATER PATIENT CENTRICITY

Whether through the use of new technologies, changes in approach to patient interaction or by making information more tailored at the individual level, personalisation is a major driver of change particularly as more providers seek to move away from cumbersome 'hospital-centric' care to 'patient-centric' support that is integrated in the wider health and social care systems: a more customer-centric approach is at the fore for many. The consensus is that if patients can be persuaded to make more use of advice based on some of the social determinants of their particular health needs, they will enjoy a better quality of life and, receive more focused health care services which can, in turn, be delivered in a cost-effective manner.[97]

The personalisation of healthcare looks set to manifest itself in many ways across different areas of the system. One example of how it may evolve is in the delivery of hospital care; rather than build bigger buildings, it seems more practical to offer treatments in a more intimate way with hospitals becoming 'smaller and more distributed' – certainly more local. Indeed, several national health systems are already preparing for an increase in walk in or 'ambulatory' out-patient care facilities, a corresponding reduction in general hospital and the establishment of more centres of excellence for complex surgery. In the UK, for example, integrating care locally is one of the key areas of focus for the NHS over the next five years.[98] Key actions on the agenda here include better integration of the varied strands of support including GPs, community nursing, mental health, social care and moving specialist care out of hospitals into the community. But joining up the primary and acute care systems relies on improved information sharing across parties and intelligent interrogation of data. In principle, in a single payer system such as the NHS this should be a credible ambition as it is more about the technological challenge than commercial interests of different parties as found in some other systems.

INTEGRATION

There are a good number of challenges to address before mass personalisation becomes a reality. The ambition is to extend access to information beyond just pills and sick-care to include behaviour and lifestyle data in the mix. So greater integration, meaning the bringing together of multiple sources of information - personal, proxy and contextual - in order to create a more holistic health profile, is vital. Delivering this will require as much policy change and collaboration between parties as it does technology development.[99] On top of this understanding data quality and differentiating between different kinds of data will also be important. As we begin to use a range of sources from accurate, complete and integrated data to, for example, circumstantial data, trying to select what is, and what is not, relevant will not be straightforward.

OWNERSHIP

End-to-end management of individuals' health only becomes possible when there is clear control, ownership or custodianship of personal health data, and that data is of high quality and consistency. Therefore, as highlighted earlier, understanding who owns what data, and who can decide who or which organisations can access it and if or how they will profit by it, is key. Failure to agree on this, some suggest could lead to a scenario where data mining and analysis will cease to be cost effective because confusion around ownership will make it hard and expensive to access. As we explore in more detail in the next section of this report, some believe that the monetization of health data is the only way to manage this process; *"in this world, only data that has monetary value will be of interest and hence supported."* But some argue that if the focus remains mainly on the financial value, then the overriding concern is that the benefits are likely to be limited to the few, targeted conditions where significant impact can be made, or to those for which the rich are willing to pay. If this problem is not sorted out many quite right, several wonder whether more individualized medicine will widen the healthcare gap rather than close it.

INDIVIDUALISED MEDICINE

It seems obvious to many that an increase in accurate information about our genes, our bodies, our behaviour and our environment can improve our understanding about personal well-being and that therefore the ability to develop and deliver more individualised medicine has great potential to shape the provision of health services in the future. A good number of those we spoke to see that within the next decade, truly bespoke, targeted healthcare at the (n=1) individual level will be available – certainly for those governments, organisations or individuals who can afford to pay. Even at a population level, many believe that precision medicine that allows decisions, treatments, practices, or products to be tailored to small groups, is a realistic ten-year ambition.

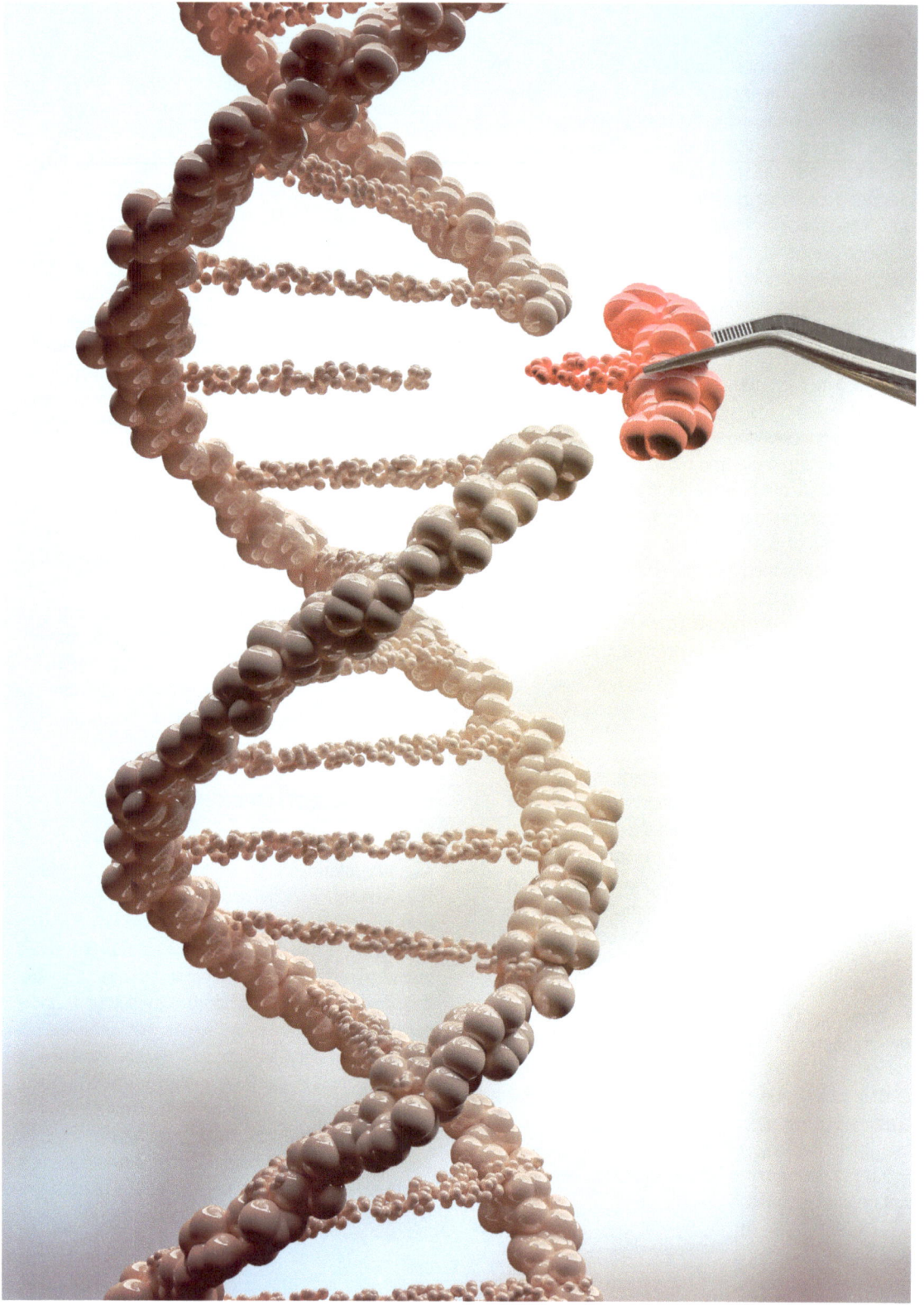

To an extent some conditions, including cancers, are already benefiting from individualised medicine. However, this is not so for the majority of cases - even though there is growing understanding of its potential. This does not necessarily mean there will be an increase in individualized treatments, rather the focus is on identifying the approaches that will be effective for specific patients based on genetic, environmental, and lifestyle factors and, as the evidence is gathered, can better inform care for an increasing number of patients. In Johannesburg the view was that *"over the next ten years, there will be constant iteration to both identify best practice and manage the market"* and that *"predictive analytics and genetic profiling together will create more connected prediction and drive hyper-personalization."*

Looking ahead most expect that personalisation will remain concentrated on specific areas, such as oncology, and that proof of impact will drive wider adoption. *"Technology will improve, and prices will drop. Medical advances will mean that the market will grow and the ability to improve prediction and manage our health accordingly will increase."* In addition, more genetic profiling will eventually reveal *"a gradual, non-linear move from reactive medicine and treatment to the delivery of preventative medicine that means we will have cheaper, faster and more effective healthcare".*

But there are reasons to be cautious. In San Francisco it was pointed out that *"15 years ago, we were talking about precision medicine which was not delivered – now it's called individualised medicine - maybe we have just changed the name."* In Johannesburg the outlook was that personalised medicine will simply be too expensive for the majority so, in poorer regions it will be a *"niche in healthcare"* and so *"for the next decade will only be for the wealthy and the rich economies."* Despite its obvious growth (see chart below), most agree that the opportunity should be kept in perspective.

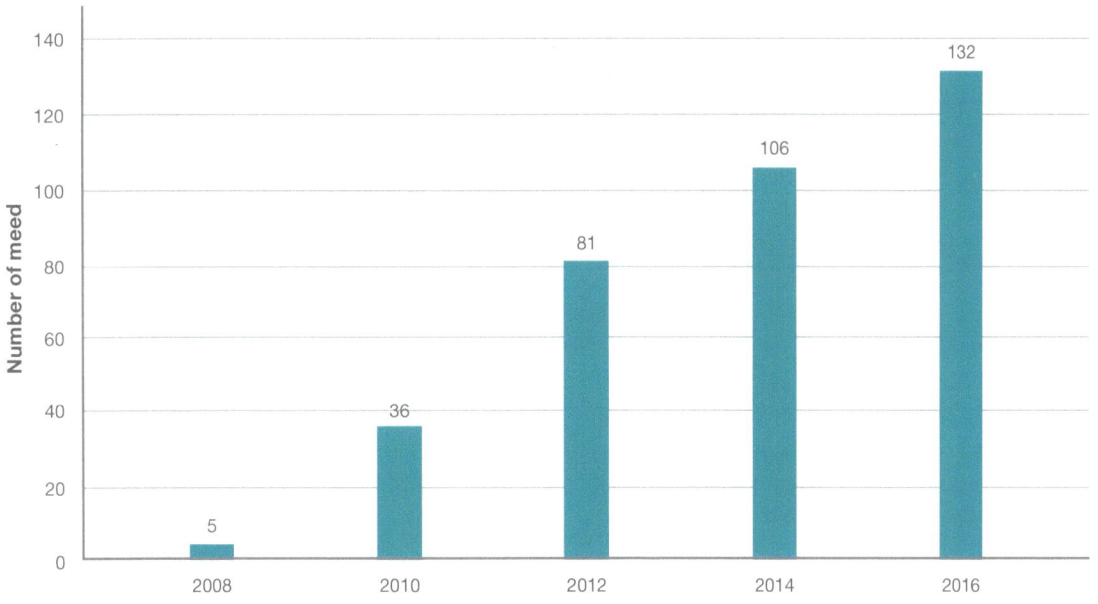

Number of Personalised Medicines (US - 2008 to 2016)

Year	Number of meed
2008	5
2010	36
2012	81
2014	106
2016	132

Source: Personalised Medicine Coalition (2017)

Many believe that personalisation will have a significant impact on the development of drugs. In Frankfurt, where a number of participants were from the pharma sector, it was suggested that individualized medicine feels *"like the end of the blockbuster era where one product would treat many thousands"* and that *"that the pharma industry needs to change, or it will not survive."* However, as is slowly being shown with some chronic conditions such as diabetes, in order to realize significant change patients will need to recognize the benefits too;[100] *"we might need to use incentives to ensure a better understanding of the patient's perspective. Without this we will not be able to have a precise diagnosis or individualized treatment."*

INDIVIDUAL BEHAVIOUR

Many believed that the greatest opportunity that personalization presents is the way it can increase public understanding around health and lifestyle; *"over the next decade we will move from patients being uninformed and dependent to becoming more informed and therefore more empowered. Certainly, they will be less encumbered by legal, social and political restrictions."*[101] In addition, as understanding of health conditions and future needs grows, it will be possible to nudge people (and systems) to change behaviour in order to prevent symptoms developing unnecessarily. Ideally this can benefit everyone. In Dubai, one scenario saw that *"as more data is increasingly easy to access at low cost we can use appropriate analysis to help improve patient behaviour."*

However, to achieve this, several major shifts need to take place:

1. **Education**: For the **patient** the focus should be on education, independent 'activation' and becoming more empowered – giving them the opportunity to use different digital tools (e.g. those provided by the likes of Atlantis Health).[102]

2. **Integration**: For the **system**, the change is about integrating multiple platforms. These include tailoring information from smart phones, wearables and biometrics etc.; delivering remote diagnostics to give accurate healthcare information; and using more AI and pattern recognition to provide personalised support, warnings and guidance of deviation from 'normal' health for you.

3. **Skills**: For **clinicians** there is a need to ensure that the use of data is not just pushed to already over stretched GPs. Properly managed, integrated data should support the provision of care and enable a more distributed supply of services.

GENOMICS

In addition to improvements in the healthcare service the widespread use of personalised data is expected to significantly reduce the cost of care. Take for example the potential from our DNA data. As the cost of genetic profiling is dropping quickly how well we use the associated information raises a number of questions. On a positive side with more investment in the sequencing of genomes, such as with the UK's Biobank[103] programme, many foresee a better understanding of "genetically defined" diseases that will aid the development of drug discovery, diagnostics and testing (see chart right). This will enable medicines to be made specifically for patient groups. As understanding of the molecular base increases, we can breakdown diseases into sub-diseases and so better treat them and even identify as yet undiagnosed conditions. But how should that information be managed by individuals, employers, insurers, healthcare providers and governments?

The Human Genome project completed the first sequence in 2003. Since then cost of profiling has reduced considerably (down from $1bn to around $100),[104] and it is now affordable and accessible through companies such as 23andme and Ancestry.com. A host of organisations such as Chinese company **iCarbonX** and Alphabet's **Verily** (see case studies) are capitalising on this and are combining biological, psychological and behavioural data, in order to provide individualized health analysis, predict users' health and so make lifestyle recommendations.

Genetic Disorders with Diagnostic Tests Available

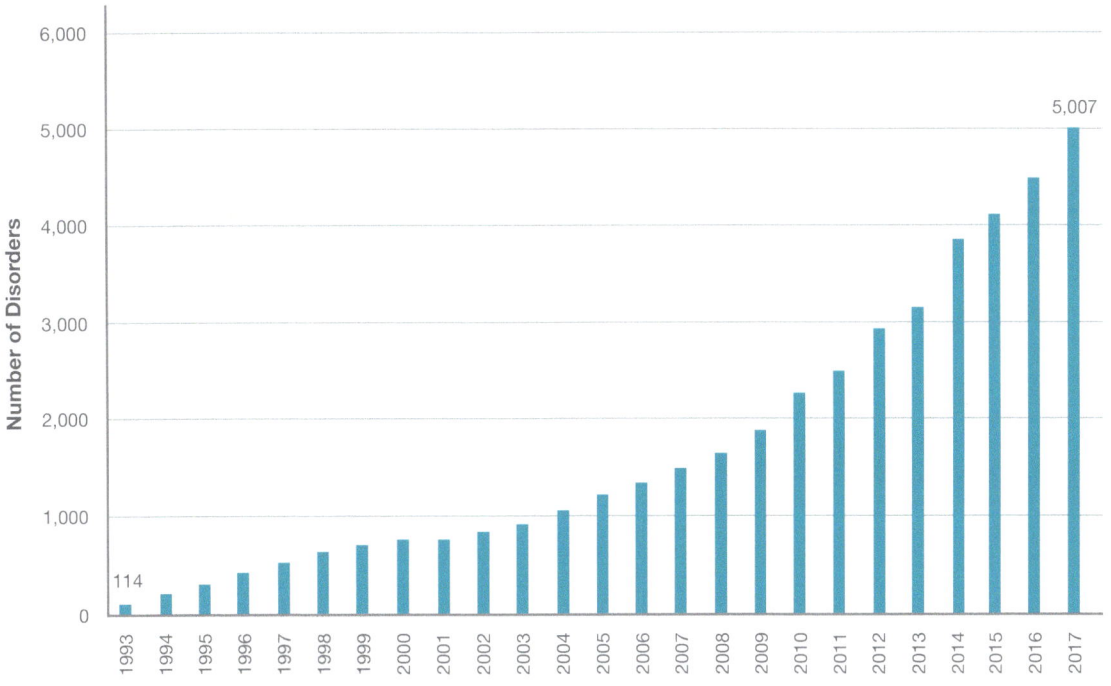

Source: Genetests (5/17)

As the cost of acquiring data declines, so the businesses around it evolve. Organisations such as **Nebula Genomics** (see case study) are changing the model so that the core genome sequence belongs to the individual but can be rented out. Genome pioneer Craig Venter's latest start-up, Human Longevity, is hugely ambitious and aims to offer genomic analysis, personalized vaccines and cell therapies, as well as supporting predictive and personalized care including cancer analysis, integrated health analysis, new-born screening and the identification of rare and undiagnosed diseases and, for a fee of $25,000 per person, wants to customize treatments for each patient's DNA.[105] Given these types of ventures it is little surprise that bioinformatics scientists and genetic counsellors are two of the fast-growing new professions.

Again, however, a word of caution, some in the US workshops felt that individualized medicine, while a bold ambition, is not going to occur universally any time soon.[106] The challenges are simply too intractable. Although some of the key ingredients are starting to align, it will take more than ten years to establish the business models that drive it, the interoperability that enables it and the insights and evidence upon which to make true impact assessments.

MICROBIOMES

Despite this there is growing support for other new technologies as, equipped with understanding of individual genetic dispositions and new intervention technologies, we can start to proactively edit genes and, for instance, undertake minimally invasive surgery thus reducing the need for major surgery in later years. Indeed, such is the enthusiasm for this, some, both in London and Mumbai, suggested that we should go beyond talking about just genetic profiling and look at the microbiomes – the genomes of our bacteria. This may well give us better, richer information about disease risk.

In Singapore it was suggested that the growth in high-resolution bio-tracking through ingestibles has led to increased innovation opportunities for smart toilets and faecal analysis. This was already highlighted as a major future opportunity area in our 2015 London 'Future of Health' event.[107] Companies such as iCarbonX in China and Japanese toilet manufacturer Toto are leaders in this area. Several platforms already analyse your urine, take your blood pressure, and send the statistics to your doctor.[108]

PERSONAL DATA STORES

Another potentially pivotal development here is the role of new personal data stores. Companies such as **digi.me** (see case study) are seeking to give control of health data 'back to the individual' and are gaining traction. US regulation now requires healthcare providers to create citizen-facing APIs while in Europe GDPR is enshrining in law greater rights for individuals to access, interrogate and correct their own data. As more patients gain 'control' of more of their health and wellness information, then they can share it, as well as other relevant personal social data, with trusted organisations. These, in turn, use this more personal information to provide more personalised health services.

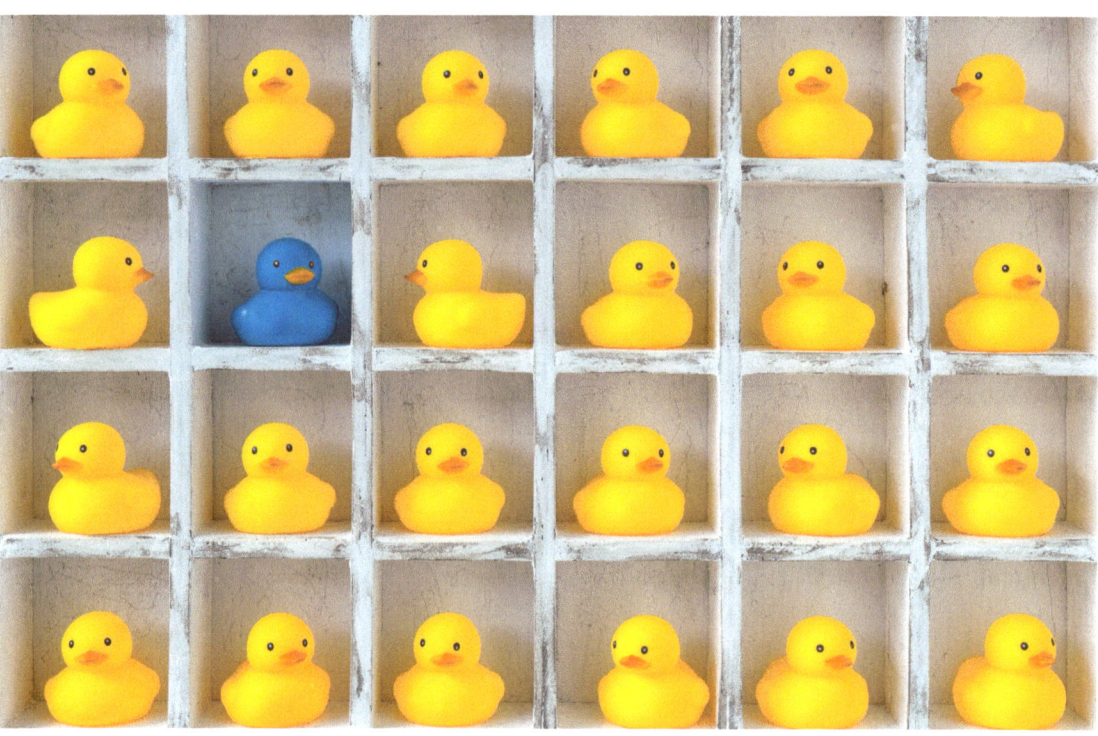

PATIENT COMMUNITIES

Core to all of this is the premise that greater shared knowledge and more peer-to-peer interaction can influence behaviour change. There is certainly evidence to support the benefits of connecting local patients (maybe digitally) who share similar symptoms. In general patients prefer to talk to others in their local community or within already known groups, so, as was highlighted in London, we should *"focus on sharing experiences within existing communities – not just in creating new ones – connecting neighbours and fellow employees who have the same conditions and so pooling people with similar characteristics with private social networks."* However, it is not a given that deeper understanding and even community support will drive behaviour change in everyone. After all, despite years of informed advice many of us still smoke - including doctors!

As more wearables and other self-managed options for data creation evolve, more lifestyle data will be linked to AI systems that will, in turn, support personalized medicine. In Singapore, a conversation was very much AI focused: *"By 2030 we see that there will be a blend of AI and human support creating the hybrid integrated healthcare system with the patient at the centre."* Chat-bot consultations, especially with pregnant women, are perhaps the most prominent example of this today but this is only just the start. Most significantly, as new tech is developed, we will have to ensure that humans become comfortable with its use so that it can be more easily deployed.

Benefits for the Patient

The tailoring of healthcare more to the individual, driven by more personal information is at the core of the future patient data ambition. If access, integration and analysis can be successfully aligned then few doubt the impact that more tailored and more focused health support can have. There may well be a few false starts, but if greater personalisation can be delivered for the many and not just the few, then the short and long-term impacts for individuals should be significant.

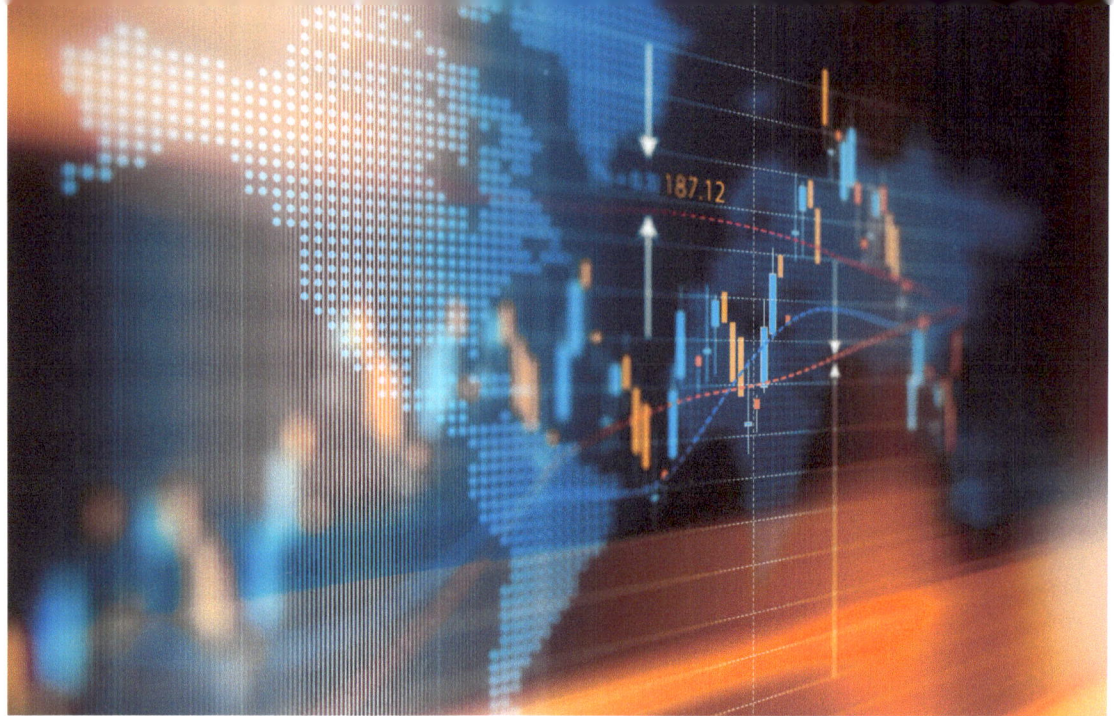

Data marketplaces

Core to considering how patient data will be accessed in the future, is its wider exchange. A key issue will be what is considered to be public commons vs. what is available for commercial use. To manage this, personal and clinical data will be represented in health data marketplaces that seek to create financial value and enable better care. Given the value of health data in some key sectors, the marketplaces will undoubtedly expand but ensuring how the patient can still benefit will be a challenge.

Along with more connected, interoperable and shared health data comes an opportunity for data marketplaces. The ability to aggregate, access and hence analyse vast amounts of patient data is a core ambition for many and achieving this through centralised systems that draw together multiple information sources is also a common wish. But there are huge costs involved and challenges around quality control. A suggested solution is to establish data marketplaces which can determine value and enable exchange. The broad view is that as *"data is a currency, it has a value and a price, so it requires a marketplace."*

EVERYTHING CONNECTED

The commonly cited view is that by 2020 the IoT will be made up of over 50bn connected devices and maybe up to 1 trillion sensors. Some see that much of this growth may well come from medical sensors that generate, track and share our health information. Indeed, the volume of health data is predicted to triple by 2020. This means that it will soon be possible to access previously inaccessible details which may have the potential to change how healthcare can be delivered. But managing this wealth of information is complicated, not least because the data needs to be cleaned and organised before it can be made available for interrogation and exchange. Also, the ordering and sharing of this will cost. How this can be achieved effectively has been the subject of much debate.

MARKETPLACES

The idea of a data marketplace is not new. Banks use data marketplace for credit-referencing: Experian is probably one of the most recognised players here. Other examples include such applications as performance analytics on mobile-operator network coverage and real-time aircraft flight information. What is new is the potential creation of multi-party data marketplaces focused specifically on healthcare which operate in a similar fashion to those in other sectors. There is much appetite for this approach and much discussion. Indeed, it was chosen as an area for deeper focus in seven of our workshops; Boston, Brussels, Dubai, Frankfurt, Johannesburg, London and Singapore. In Boston, the concept was articulated as *"a way to capture the inherent value of patient data and more easily allocate it and share it among the players, rather than just letting it accrue to those collecting it today."* Some felt they offer *"an important step in building relationships with patients (raising awareness of the value of their data could help) and in helping patients change their behaviour."* All agreed that there are some pivotal decisions that must be addressed when establishing such marketplaces include governance models and whether, for instance, they are independent platforms or limited ownership hybrids. Answering these questions and working out how to manage patient data exchange is an area that many organisations are currently exploring.

McKinsey sees that data marketplaces are "platforms that connect providers and consumers of data sets and data streams, ensuring high quality, consistency, and security. The data suppliers authorize the marketplace to license their information on their behalf, following defined terms and conditions. Consumers can play a dual role by providing data back to the marketplace."[109] Here, key enablers include; the building of an ecosystem, opening up new monetization opportunities, enabling crowdsourcing, supporting interoperability, creating a central point of 'discoverability' and achieving consistent data quality. Data marketplaces differ from data warehouses in that they allow for cataloguing and curating.[110] Although most traditionally begin within a single company or organisation, it is when they start to connect across a wider ecosystem that they prove to be an effective platform for information sharing and analysis – and hence create value.

HEALTH DATA MARKETPLACES

Some patient data is already being traded - but as yet largely only on a bilateral company-to-company basis. Indeed, many would argue that 'private' data marketplaces have been around in the healthcare sector for a while – particularly within or serving the pharmaceutical and insurances industries. IQVIA, for example, is one of the more well-known organisations that have been built on the ability to acquire, analyse and then sell health data - especially around clinical development trials.[111] Their success and that of others led several experts to comment that *"perhaps health data is a gold-mine?"* Certainly, it has *"very high potential value"* and if used responsibly could drive significant change, maybe even paying for basic healthcare.[112]

Going forward it was widely agreed that *"ecosystems for trading data are already emerging and personal and clinical data will be represented in these new healthcare data marketplaces."* Many suggest that the process will become more open and transparent as more organisations seek to combine multiple patient data sets. Ensuring trust in the system is vital to its survival so there was concern that due consideration should to be given to the fundamental principles behind the establishment of a marketplace and much debate about what these should be. Everyone also agreed that different business models still need to be explored to establish "how a data marketplace can pay for itself" and *"what is the sustainable model for data trading?"* A number of existing open data platforms were discussed - including the Genome project and the UK biobank. All agreed that this is work in progress, *"there will be business models that will be trustworthy, but we haven't seen them yet."*

While there is a cadre of established companies which are active in the development of healthcare data marketplaces including TCS, IBM and Alphabet (via Verily and DeepMind), it is also an area of high start-up activity with many seeking to integrate AI and block-chain.[113,114,115,116] In addition a number of organisations are taking different approaches to data ownership, for example:

- **HealthVerity** provides a marketplace for data providers and data buyers.[117] This has "linkable HIPAA-compliant, de-identified healthcare data on more than 300m individuals in the U.S. from more than 30 national healthcare data suppliers." That means the marketplace includes data from medical claims, prescription claims, lab results, electronic medical records and other data sources.[118] Its, founders advocate the potential for researchers to undertake deeper exploration of data that could, for example, provide a better understanding of disease progression and a drug's impact through the course of a disease.

- **CoverUs** sees that "your health care data should be your private property, and if anyone is making money from that data, it should be you" and is focused on rebalancing the 'billions of dollars' that private companies make by selling individuals medical data.[119] The system provides users with a digital wallet that is accessible from their smartphone. This can then be populated by data from their electronic health record, wearable devices and other health trackers which can then be shared, and indeed monetized, by the individual, whether it's with their healthcare provider, medical researchers or other sources.[120] The offering rests upon a proprietary cryptocurrency which is earned by sharing data.

PERSONAL VS. ANONYMOUS DATA

Most agree that these and increasingly sophisticated data marketplaces will be a key feature of the future of healthcare and that many will be driven by more and better-quality patient data. As this evolves, so too will the need for a clear demarcation between personal data and anonymous data. At the moment, most of the data being exchanged is aggregated or anonymized, but there were questions around whether this will always be the case. Consent is the key issue here. Lessons may well be taken from, for instance, CODE - the European collaboration on oncology data[121] which proposes there needs to be deeper consideration of what is meant by meaningful consent in the digital economy so that citizens understand how their personal data could be used; and where they can decide what happens to it.[122] Not everyone agreed that this is an area of significant public concern pointing out that *"people say they are worried about data but they will sell it for less than a penny."*

In South Africa several consider that *"there ought to be publicly managed global health data exchanges that ensure that high quality information is made available for all key parties."* Given the sensitivity of the topic effective regulation is clearly important. In Singapore the argument was that broader public awareness is key to ensuring that the maximum benefits of data marketplaces are realised - *"If the data value extraction can be democratised then this will open the door to information sharing at an extraordinary scale."* There was also much discussion about how this can be achieved; one view in Canada was that *"people like rewards – using air miles as an incentive for healthy living is working."* Others took a more holistic approach pointing out that *"in the healthcare market, trust, consent and governance are the first challenges to address ahead of building the marketplace and the products that can operate within it."*[123]

In the Brussels event, legal expertise considered that *"there should be a clear demarcation of what is the commons space vs. the commercial space"* and that *"if health data is to be exchanged in a marketplace, regulatory frameworks should be developed that determine how we build / incentivise reward systems for investment, trading and stewardship."*[124] Moreover *"there has to be clear governance and comprehensive guidance on both accountability and quality of data as well as views on who will use the data and what they will actually pay for."*

In London, there were fundamental questions around what marketplaces are used for and whether they act as mechanisms for social good or are a way of monetizing human failure. These included:

- How can you define what is to be used and not used?
- How do you define a marketplace – is it a co-operative?
- Who will define what the commons space is vs. the commercial space?

And before we forget the practicalities when all these challenges are sorted out, many agree that *"someone still has to manage the process so that the all-important data to be 'cleaned' and that someone will have to be paid for their efforts."*[125] In some discussions it was apparent that not all consider that data marketplaces will be a good thing. In South Africa, the position was

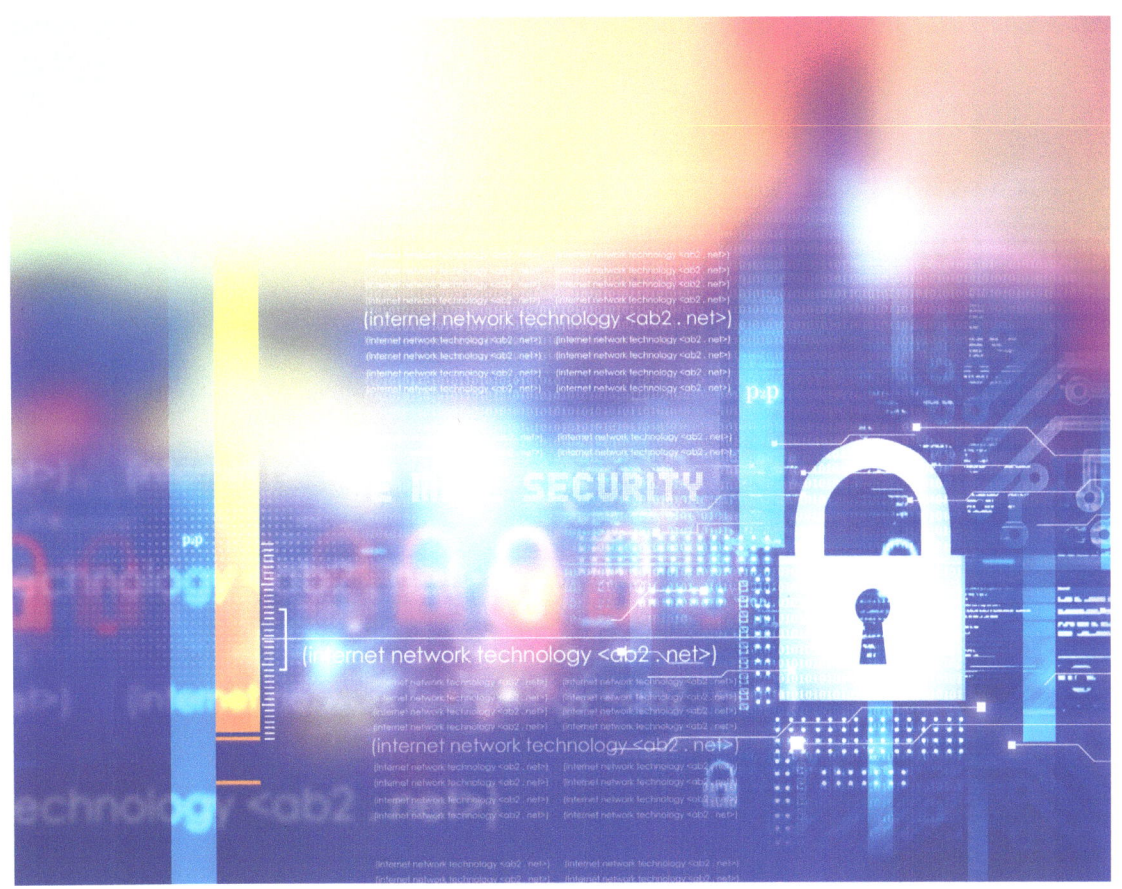

that *"healthcare data should not be monetised. It should be seen a public good and used to benefit all. Specifically, it should not be in the hands of a few private companies nor should it be a source of profit."* Others see a parallel with the different opt-in vs opt-out approaches used around the world with organ donation – putting the choice of benefit in the hands of the patient.

However, in Frankfurt, the final assessment was that new marketplaces will emerge based on business models that offer greater incentives for success and penalties for failure. By 2025 we will have clearer views about which data we should use for what purpose. *"As patients become more supportive, driven by disruptors such as Apple, Facebook, Amazon they will be prepared to buy and sell their data, so it is important to understand what they will be willing to share."* That said, some consider that there will have to be a paradigm shift in behaviours and that data markets will only work if patients understand the process: *"We have to make data marketplaces simple."* To achieve this there needs to be more research around health and prevention and greater health literacy; payment needs to be based on outcomes and pharmaceutical companies in particular will have to sell 'better health' not 'managing sickness'. Furthermore, the transparency that will required from data market places will drive greater awareness around efficacy so it may well be that in future, alongside treating disease, doctors will be reimbursed for training people to remain healthy.

Benefits for the Patient

Patient data is already being traded, albeit at an aggregated and anonymised level, but this is not widely recognised. As awareness grows and there is greater focus on more personalised information, a common question is the extent to which individuals will be involved in managing their personal data and whether they will be able to benefit from it financially. There are issues around privacy and trust, but maybe well-designed models with a greater focus on the social and health / wellness benefits, as well as the financial side, could develop. Given the rising value of health data, marketplaces will undoubtedly expand but ensuring that the patient gains advantage will be pivotal.

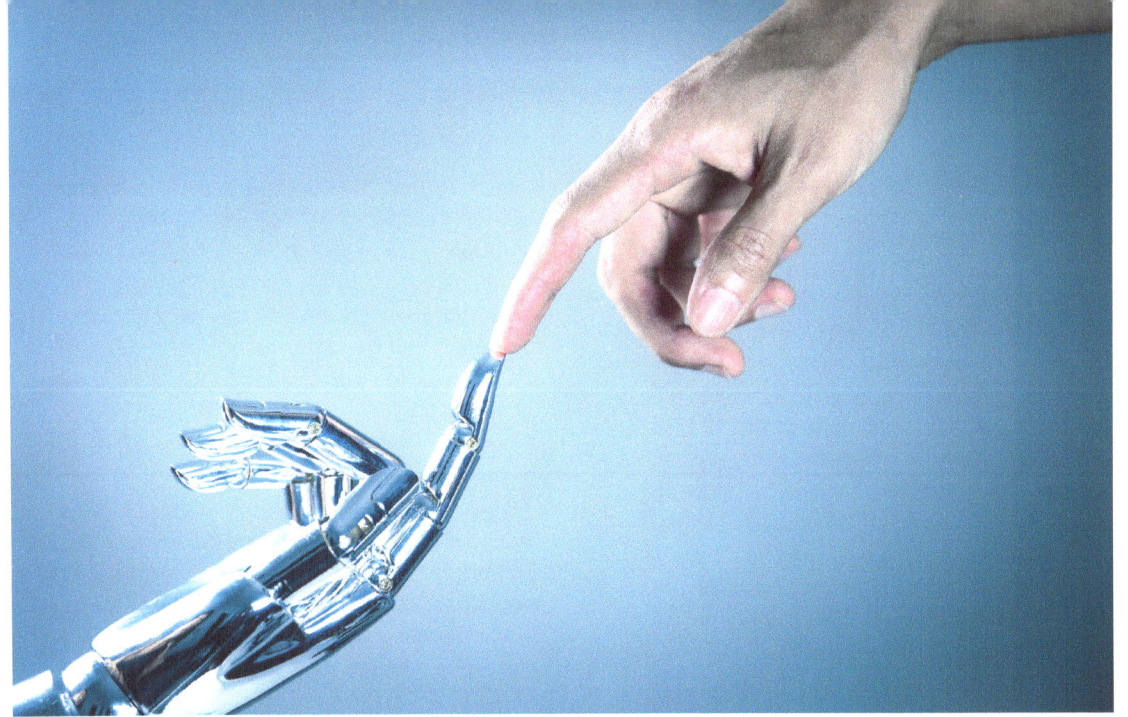

The impact of AI

Initial advances from machine learning and pattern recognition will be significant in enabling more efficient diagnosis and better prediction. As deep learning and self-learning then develop, the ability to deal with unstructured data delivers major improvements in diagnosis and treatment and AI is embedded into many clinical decisions. Moreover, with voice and facial recognition increasingly analysing users' behaviour patterns, AI is also applied to identify stress and anxiety.

Today we can see growing activity across the AI arena – barely a day goes by without a new report or media feature on how AI will take over and replace our jobs or else deliver massive improvements in efficiency across multiple sectors. From energy management and traffic flows to education and healthcare, investment in new AI propositions is growing rapidly.

The potential impact of AI on healthcare is considered to be enormous – and most believe that much of this revolves around the improved analysis of patient data. An initial perspective that *"as more people use AI health advice, the more data is collected and therefore the more accurate diagnosis can be"* was widely supported. However, it was often pointed out that the impact of AI will be far greater than just this. *"We are just at the very early stages"* was the common view.

INITIAL GROWTH OF AI

AI is already making primary care more effective and efficient. This potential has been frequently reported by the likes of IBM Watson[126] and Google Deep Mind[127,128,129]. Another player Babylon Health[130,131,132] has recently struck a deal with Chinese internet giant Tencent to provide an automated symptom-checker and paid-for video consultations to WeChat's almost 1bn users. At the same time in India Tricog[133] is improving the time, cost and efficiency of cardiac diagnosis,[134] highlighting immunotherapy cancer links[135] and identifying rare diseases in children lacking key enzymes. Elsewhere artificial intelligence (AI) is being trained by a unit of Alphabet, to identify cancerous tissues and retinal damage. Other notable AI healthcare companies include CloudMedx, iCarbonX, Deep Genomics, Lunit and Zephyr Health,[136] and, in an adjacent space of meditation, the latest version of Headspace.[137] As patients' data is collected from smartphones and "wearables", they will teach AIs to do much more. Future AIs will, for instance, provide automated medical diagnosis from a description of your symptoms, spot behavioural traits that suggest you are at particular risk of a specific condition and even work out if you are suffering from depression.

In Oslo, the observation was that *"AI adoption will be led by primary care support with a particular focus on specialist conditions."* In Dubai, the perspective was that we are *"very much in the learning phase"* but that within 10 years the impact can be significant. In Brussels, although concern was expressed about how 'clean' the data needs to be for it to have impact in the short term, it was suggested that, while initial focus is on improving diagnosis, *"over time we will quickly move to using AI for treatment."*

PATTERN RECOGNITION

Until now many of the developments in the news have been niche applications. For instance, while **Deep Mind** (see case study) has been in the headlines with its pioneering work in machine learning, as yet most of its healthcare activity with the NHS in the UK has focused on leveraging more mature pattern recognition via the Streams technology in a few specific areas. These include acute kidney injury with the Royal Free and age-related macular degeneration in partnership with Moorfields Eye Hospital. However, as it and other organisations gain access to more medical data, the potential from pattern recognition alone is seen to be massive. *"At the moment, the focus is on imaging and radiology because that is well structured information and good for pattern detection."* In these first steps the dependency on restricting usage to high quality, clean data sets has both pros and cons. On the positive side it is allowing swift and successful proof of capability, but, on the other hand, the range of patient data currently available for analysis is, in some eyes, relatively narrow.

"AI is already having impact where we have structured data available – and so can improve efficiency."[138] For example, DeepMind has crunched data from thousands of retinal scans to train an AI algorithm to detect signs of eye disease more quickly and efficiently than human specialists. However, if it is going to have wider effect, then either AI will have to become adept at dealing with unstructured data or new ways must be found to clean data before it can be fed into the system. Achieving this will rely on a combination of regulatory standards and new business models around reimbursement that make the effort worthwhile. Key will be the role in helping with the integration of multiple sources of information. *"If we get it right there could be a different 'geometry of connection' based on human relationships."*[139]

Recognising that so far this is largely about machines doing what humans can do, but faster and with increasing accuracy, the overall consensus was that in the short-term machine learning and pattern recognition will support doctors – and certainly not replace them: *"Doctors diagnose accurately 74% of the time."*[140] An agreed view was that *"AI is already here – we are using algorithms already and learning from them. AI is improving research effectiveness, increasing the efficiency of clinical care and enhancing education."* AI and doctors are increasingly working together.

ARTIFICIAL GENERAL INTELLIGENCE

Although we are still in the early days, the possible future change that can be achieved with the use of AI with patient data is universally seen as being substantial. Within the wealth of potential AI opportunities being explored, in Boston it was suggested that it is important to recognize that:

- AI can be applied across a broad spectrum of healthcare provision including R&D, care delivery, patient engagement and behavioural modification, population health, admin and material resource planning.[141]

- Moreover, assumptions are being made on the *"key characteristics of future AI in healthcare will be that it is ambient, global, open-sourced, patient-focused and include humans in the loop."*

Several experts in London and the US pointed out that while some are talking about the ambition for AI as Artificial General Intelligence (where a machine that could successfully perform any intellectual task that a human being can), others are looking way beyond that target. One side-remark in Boston was that *"my ideal view of this is Scarlet Johansen in the movie HER – is that the ultimate AI experience?"* 'She' is intuitive, sensitive and playful.

In a positive scenario from London, the perspective was that in the next decade *"AI increasingly automates routines that currently occupy up to 80% of the GP's time. In doing so it enhances human interactions, drives development of regulation, thereby reducing revisits and rewiring decision making."* Doctors can then focus on more of the 'human' activities so *"AI will lead to a change in the relationship between providers and patients."* Others suggested that *"we will move from isolated pilots to established solutions for single diseases and then on to holistic approaches. Over time algorithms will build trust and lead to much greater efficiencies in diagnosis and the management of disease progression."*[142]

AI IN CHINA

It was often highlighted - and especially in Singapore, Dubai and India - that although much of the media attention is on US and UK based enterprises, we should be paying closer attention to what is underway in China. Recent analysis by the Economist (see chart on the next page) highlights this and argues that China may well beat America at AI.[143] Over the past decade, while the number of AI based patent applications in the US has risen by 25%, albeit coming from a lower base those from Chinese companies has doubled. Moreover, as of the end of 2016, with 7,000 organisations in operation, China had the world's second largest portfolio of AI companies. With 730m Internet users, some see China as the *"Saudi Arabia of data"* providing massive amounts of rich information for new algorithms to experiment with. Within healthcare, as it seeks to build a full 'digital life ecosystem' **iCarbonX** (see case study) is just one of the Chinese companies getting significant investment support and is one of the fastest growing in the sector.

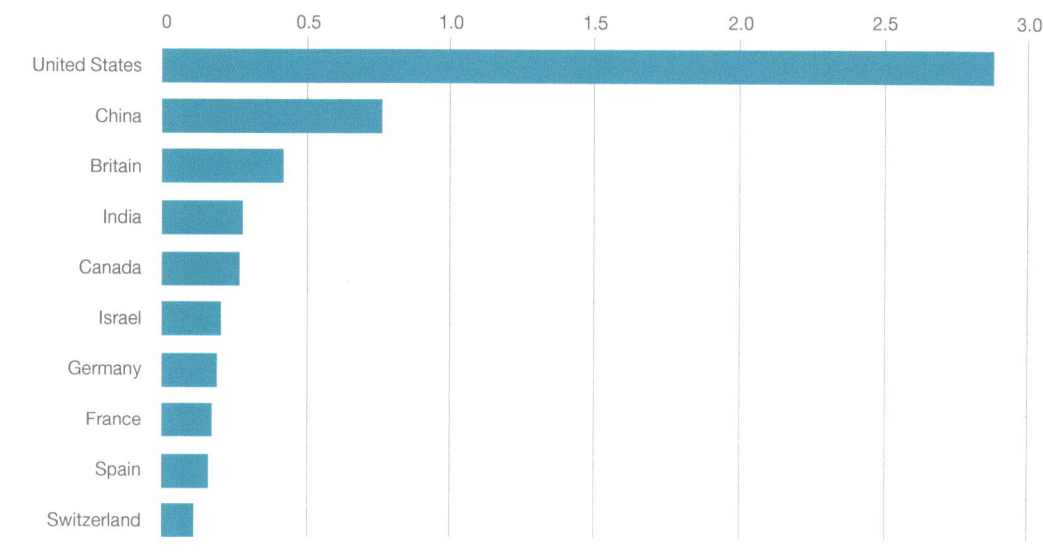

Number of Artifical-Intelligence Companies
Selected countries, 2016,'000

Source: Economist.com 2017

DEEP, SELF AND REINFORCED LEARNING

As we shift from pattern recognition and machine learning to deep-learning, self-learning and reinforced learning, the view in Singapore, was that, *"by 2030, AI will be embedded in much clinical decision support providing greater precision and personalization for patients and higher productivity for clinicians - all reinforced by more automated work flows."* For the consumer, new apps will become more clinically focused which will facilitate medical decision making. For hospitals (and healthcare providers), med-tech will incorporate more AI into equipment for detection and prediction. It was also suggested that as we shift to reinforced learning - where AI agents learn by trial and error from their own actions and experiences and so take actions to maximise some notion of cumulative reward - then we can really be more efficient in the data we use. *"The next stage of AI will require less not more data. As we move to self-learning, machines will not have to sift through lots of information and the amount of data needed to be processed will decrease – machines will know exactly what to look for and focus on that key data."* Then, as AI develops 'soft-skills' *"we can spend less time collecting data and more time connecting the dots and conceptually thinking about the problems."*

In the US one view was that AI will have particular impact both at a national population level (resource optimization, machine vision, model development etc.), but also at an individual level. *"Nationally the initial focus will include data brokerage and government domains but will then move onto example applications such as micro insurance where pricing, incentivisation and guarantees will all occur at an individual level."* There will be a growing need for regulation that, as with all new technologies, will have to strike a balance between helping to accelerate innovation but at the same time manage its ethical implementation and implication. Getting this right will open the door to many more personal applications that will aid the patient and the healthcare professional. In the first instance these are likely to be around *"the provision of routine applications however the continued growth in mass-personalization will most likely drive outcomes based on patient preferences rather than physician preferences."*

AI AND MENTAL HEALTH

Looking forward, several also commented on the implications of greater integration of Alexa, Siri and similar voice activated platforms. As these services develop, we may unlock the ability to sense and analyse individual behaviour patterns and consequently deliver a wider range of AI-driven support. One specific example that gained traction across the discussions is the use of emerging technologies in diagnosing anxiety and supporting mental health. In many of our conversations the view was that *"mental health is a growing issue that has not been getting the right level of attention in patient data discussions."* This may be changing as it was also observed that *"facial recognition software[144] already has the capacity to recognise stress and anxiety and, alongside other digital diagnostic tools - such as voice pattern analysis, it will be increasingly used to identify and monitor mental health problems."* Many believed that this might herald a step change in the way mental health could be diagnosed and treated. **Facebook** (see case study), for example is seeking to make a contribution to the mental health arena using AI analytics of Instagram feeds to diagnose depression. Although there are obvious benefits to this, in Dubai questions were raised around the negative implications if more detailed information about patients' mental health became available, *"if the information is available to them, will employers refuse to recruit people who may be prone to depression?"*

In some circumstances AI and chat-bots give those who are uncomfortable talking to others the confidence to communicate more openly because they have a perceived anonymity. This has proved to be successful in Singapore, where *"mental health is not as openly discussed as it ought to be"*. Initial papers[145] detailing evidence of the potential of chat-bots for mental health care have started to explore this and the role of technology in 'emotional chatting.' Elsewhere chat-bots are being used to help with depression.[146] Also in Singapore chat-bots are an increasingly popular source of information and advice for pregnant women who, in a deeply conservative culture, often find it difficult to be open and honest with human doctors. Technology such as this is not only felt to be less judgmental, but it is convenient too; there is no need to make appointments and the conversation can take place from patient's homes at their time of choosing rather than in a surgery which some may find too public. In Mumbai comments reinforced the view that AI can support diagnosis of mental health[147] and also socially unacceptable diseases such as tuberculosis where *"people often lie about whether there is TB in their household."*

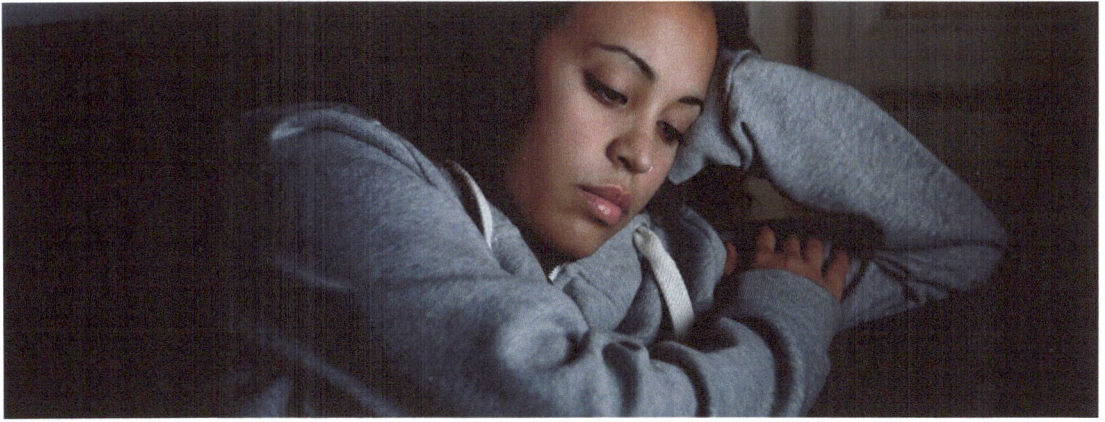

Although AI can release humans from mundane tasks and enable them to work on more exciting and value-added tasks it is not without risk and indeed most would argue it comes with its own set of responsibilities. Indeed, it was clear through our conversations, that human evil, incompetence and poor design remain a big threat for the foreseeable future. There are concerns that although AI technology alone may not reveal any inherent biases, it may unleash all manner of biases that reflect those of the humans who design the systems. Given this there is a growing sense that AI should be used not just for the right predictions, but also to make predictions for the right reasons. While AI is on a par with humans in aspects such as reading radiology images, the same neural network algorithms have potential for discriminatory profiling based on facial recognition and other decisions that have implications for society – potentially showing racial or ageist bias for example. *"What if algorithms present different treatment decisions about patients depending on their age, sex, race or even insurance status or ability to pay?"* Given this, some argue regulators should step up and ensure that tech companies and manufacturers be held liable for the misuse of their AI-enabled products in the same way that pharmaceutical firms are responsible for the harmful side-effects of their drugs. This needs to be taken seriously as retro-fitting effective principles will be like shutting Pandora's box. However, a recent Financial Times article pointed out that there are estimated to be just 100 researchers in the western world grappling with the ethics of AI in healthcare. That seems far too few, given the scale of the challenge.[148]

Of course, having the data and the AI capability doesn't guarantee improved quality or reduced costs in health care. Intervention models and care plans also need to be in place. Some argue that in an era of high-volume and high-velocity, real-time data, these limitations will slow the adoption. Given the ethical challenges perhaps this would not be entirely a bad thing. And yet, across multiple areas of healthcare, it is evident that the enthusiasm for AI to make a major contribution is growing apace. There are tangible results from its early use and as the technology and societal acceptance evolves, it seems that the future potential in indeed discernible.

Benefits for the Patient

Discussion of the impact of AI is pervasive and the potential for change is substantial. If patients are willing to both engage with new systems and also provide more of their personal data for analysis, the capability for earlier diagnosis and hence treatment is increasingly palpable. While trust is a pivotal issue, the possibility of faster, more effective healthcare support may also be on the horizon.

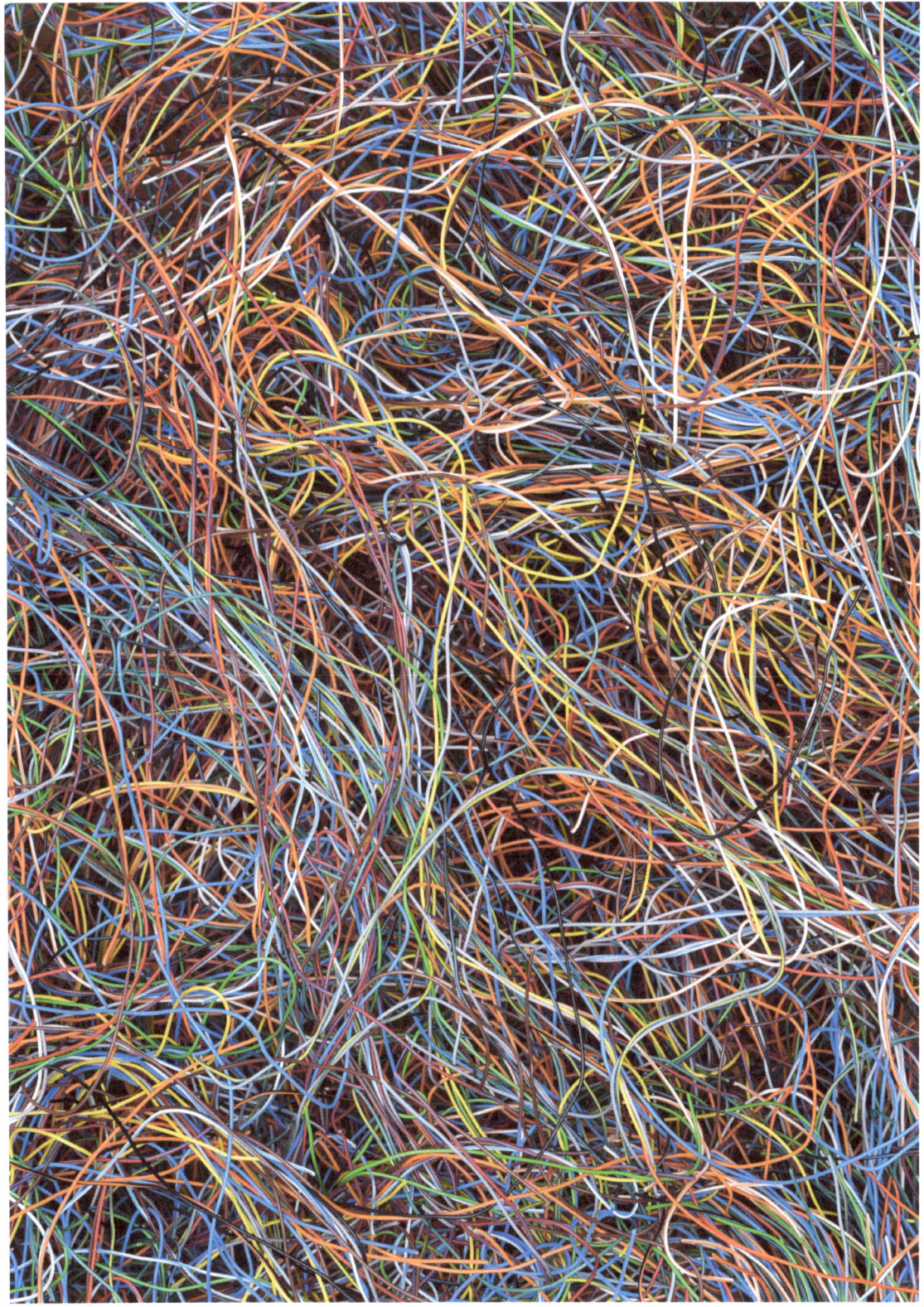

CASE STUDY:

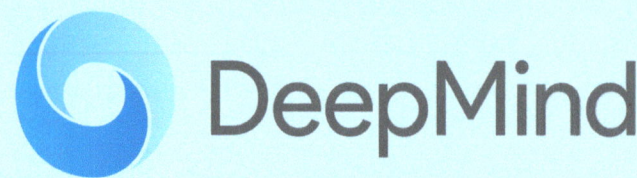

Founded in 2010 in London and acquired by Google for £400m four years later, Deep Mind has been one of the most visible of the world's AI companies – largely through its success in building machine learning algorithms that can beat the best in the world at Go. Its rather bold ambition is to "solve intelligence, (and) use it to make the world a better place." DeepMind, together with Amazon, Google, Facebook, IBM, and Microsoft, is a founding member of Partnership on AI, an organisation devoted to the society-AI interface. While DeepMind is not exclusively a healthcare company, its products with the clearest path to commercialisation are focused here. As such, led by co-founder Mustafa Suleyman, the DeepMind Health business[149] is one of its most public activities as the company seeks to bring its leading expertise to bear on the health sector and its choice to initially do this with the UK's NHS which offers a single, standardised market. It is collaborating with the UK's National Health Service on delivering better care for conditions that affect millions of people worldwide.[150]

DeepMind has partnerships with four large hospital groups to which it provides its best-known healthcare product - an app called Streams. This is designed to decrease the incidence of acute kidney injury before it occurs by alerting clinicians to the warning signs that indicate a patient is a candidate for such an injury. The app itself doesn't yet contain any deep learning AI at present but it is likely elements will make their way into the products in future. With other NHS partnerships DeepMind has been testing whether its products can analyse medical scans more quickly than doctors.

If the pilots prove successful, DeepMind can provide the software as a means of cutting down doctors'

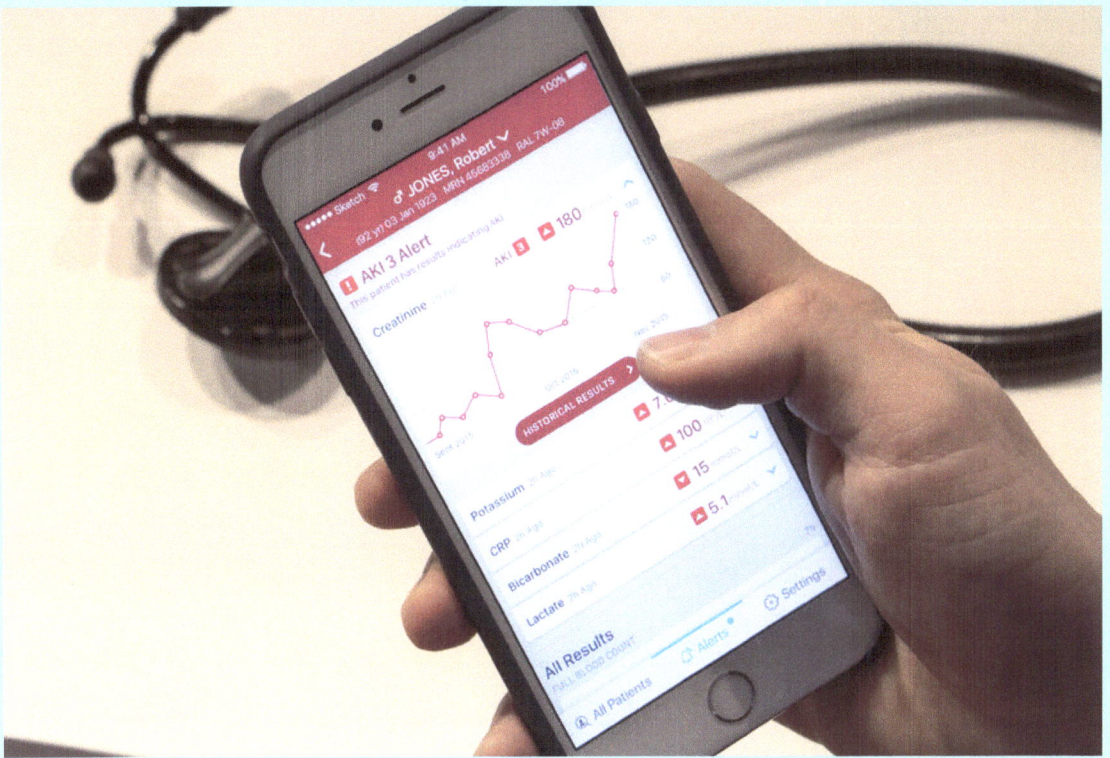

busy work, so they can get on with seeing and treating patients.[151] Although facing a legal push-back from the way the data from 1.6m patients was shared by the Royal Free NHS Trust in 2015 during the co-development of Streams,[152] it is now rolling out further collaborations including with the Taunton and Somerset NHS Foundation Trust, where it uses pattern recognition to "alert doctors and nurses to a potential deterioration in their patients' vital signs that could indicate a serious problem." The app is available at the bedside to alert doctors and nurses to any patients needing immediate assessment and help them rapidly determine whether the patient has other serious conditions such as acute kidney injury.[153] Results are impressive with nurses triaging patients in less than 30 seconds compared to the norm of up to four hours. "This is really based on the patient, so that what we've got in there is data about the patient and about what's happening to the patient while they're here with us as an in-patient that can help us identify when there are potential problems." It is a fully integrated EPR with DeepMind acting as the data processor and delivering that EPR via a mobile application. In other collaborations, DeepMind, Moorfields Hospital and two London universities are trying to see if AI software can learn to read OCT retina pictures, head and neck images and mammography scans as well as or better than doctors.[154]

Initially, DeepMind is not making money from its NHS collaboration. "Only when we can prove that we have improved outcomes will we be paid accordingly within IT supplier market rates. We're not driven by a desire to maximize profit, but rather to create a mutually sustainable business model."[155] As such, DeepMind is 'years away' from major healthcare revenues. In 2016 it reported a loss of £94m. However, with its pioneering research in deep learning, all its health data, strong partnerships with the NHS and deep pockets of Alphabet, few doubt that DeepMind will be one of the companies changing the way people experience health care.

CASE STUDY:

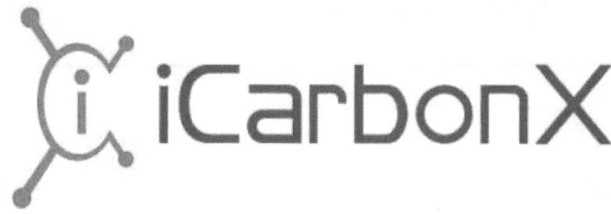

Within the fast-growing Chinese AI community that is part of the country's ambition to be a global leader by 2030, there is one healthcare company that is already standing out on the global stage. While many other of the high-profile Chinese start-ups are focused on facial recognition and driverless cars, one of the leaders is very much seeking to change healthcare.

Only founded in 2015, iCarbonX (ICX) has quickly become one of the fastest growing AI companies in the sector. Having already received over $600m in funding and now officially a 'unicorn' it tops many charts[156] and is making strong headway in its ambition to build a 'digital life ecosystem' combining biological, psychological and behavioural data, provide individualized health analysis, predict users' future health and so make recommendations on everything from diet to exercise. The company uses the analogy of providing a roadmap "that shows us where we are in terms of our health, with clear place markers for risks and opportunities. A guide based on the experience of those on the road ahead that gives signals about which paths lead to health, or to disease. A compass that points where to step first. All in a GPS that makes it easier to move toward our personal health goals, every day."[157]

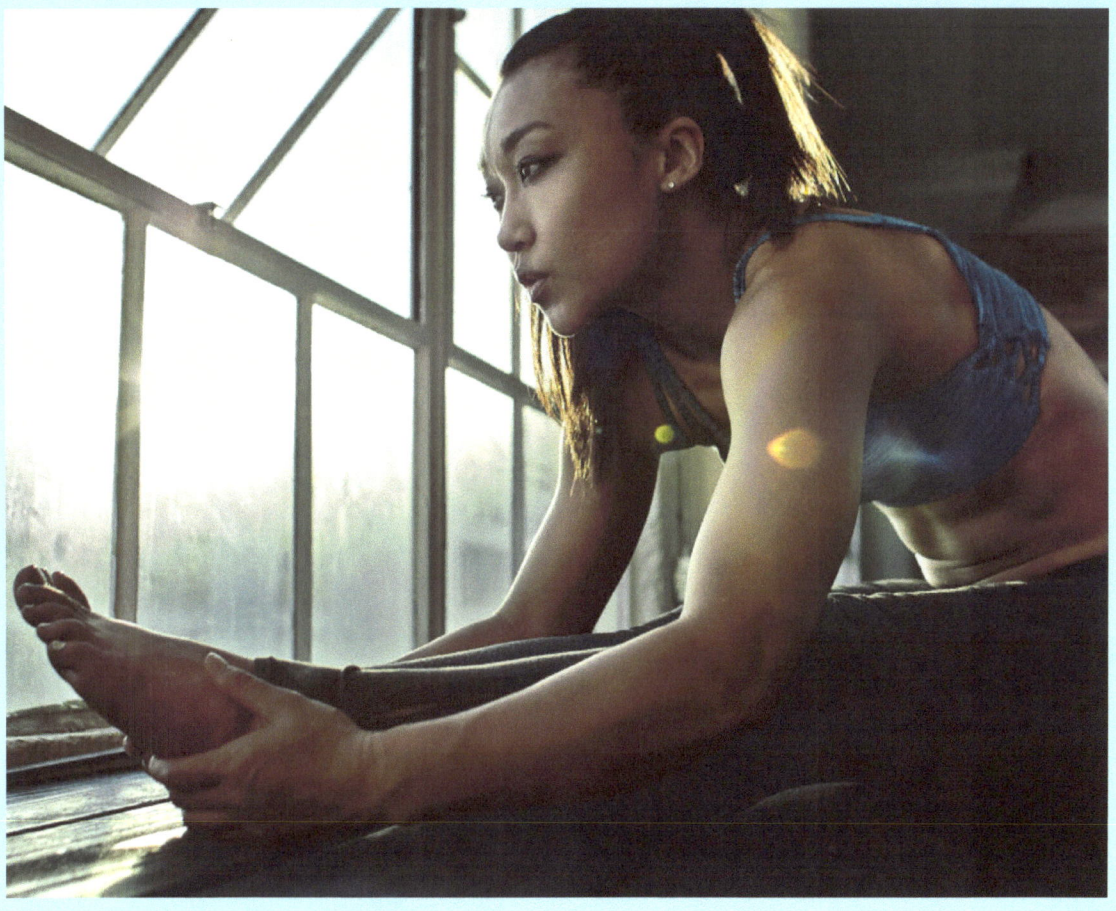

ICX wants to capture more intelligence about your body than has ever before been possible. Starting with your DNA profile and adding fit-bit style activity and key health information plus frequent blood tests, heart data and your medical history, the goal is "continuous monitoring of your health and suggestions of adjustments you might make in your diet and behaviour before you slip from being healthy into the early stages of an illness."[158] Integrating data fed from a broadening range of sources including partners such as Patientslikeme, Sema4 and HealthTell is an AI system that undertakes the core analysis. Founded by Jun Wang, former professor at the University of Copenhagen and founder of the Beijing Genomics Institute, ICX recognises that this is 'ridiculously complicated'. However, in blending Chinese AI expertise with global health data sources the ambition is to quickly move from working with populations in the tens of millions required to get meaningful insights towards far greater population sets. Starting in China with plenty of people and less stringent privacy laws than some regions, patient data is already being gained from a growing range of feeds including faecal analysis and continuous heart monitoring. Aiming at a target $200 for an AI-generated personal full profile, ICX sees that it can make a major contribution to preventative activities and bringing down the cost of health care globally.

CASE STUDY:

facebook.

Facebook is already widely used by clinical trial recruiters. This is a growing revenue stream for the company with some forecasting a health-sector spend of $3.1 billion on digital advertising by 2020.[159] There are millions of health groups on Facebook where people with a variety of health conditions discuss their symptoms. But, so far, many marketers have not been using that data in their outreach. This is now changing as the company formalises patient groups so that, despite recent public revelations about personal information misuse, pharmaceutical companies become more confident in data integrity.[160] This is intended to drive a change in the platform's cut of a growing direct to consumer ad spend in a sector where the digital share is currently only 3%.

However, it is not just in targeting patients that Facebook is becoming more active in healthcare. Another big future bet is on making a positive impact on mental health. Although frequently criticised for detrimental effects, especially on heavy users,[161] the company is using AI to monitor its customers' online behaviour for patterns which indicate depression, and to reach out in an effort to prevent suicide. For example, photos on Instagram can signal depression, depending on the colours they contain, the times at which they are posted and whether they show faces.[162] 2017 Harvard research has showed that Instagram can help diagnose depression better than your GP.[163] Machine learning tools successfully identified markers of depression from participant Instagram photos, using colour analysis, metadata components, and algorithmic face detection with "resulting models outperformed general practitioners' average unassisted diagnostic success rate for depression."[164] Facebook is now expected to incorporate the analysis within its platform to provide new avenues for early screening and detection of mental illness. As social networks come under increasing pressure on trust and truth, how effectively this is managed is being watched by many across healthcare.

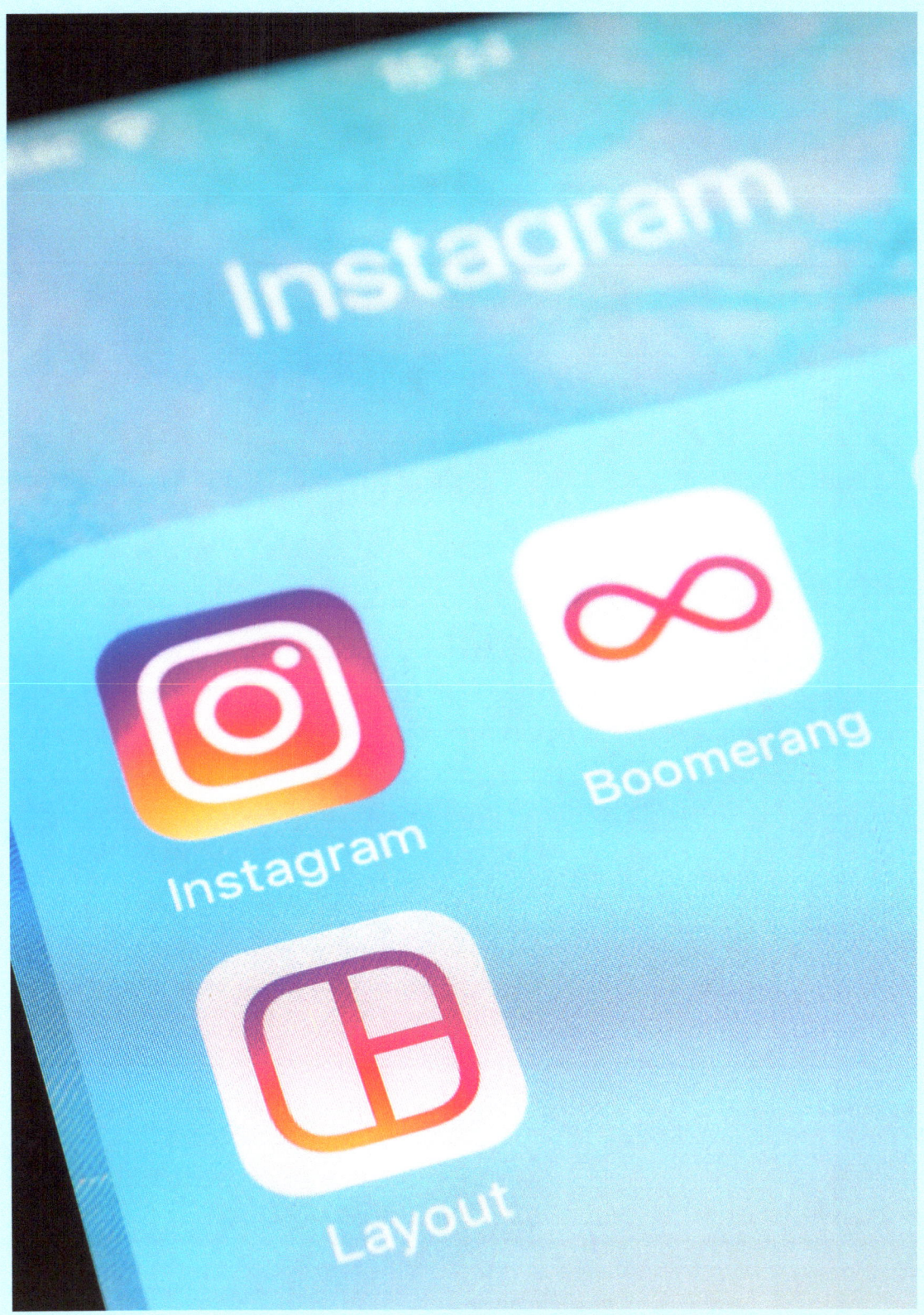

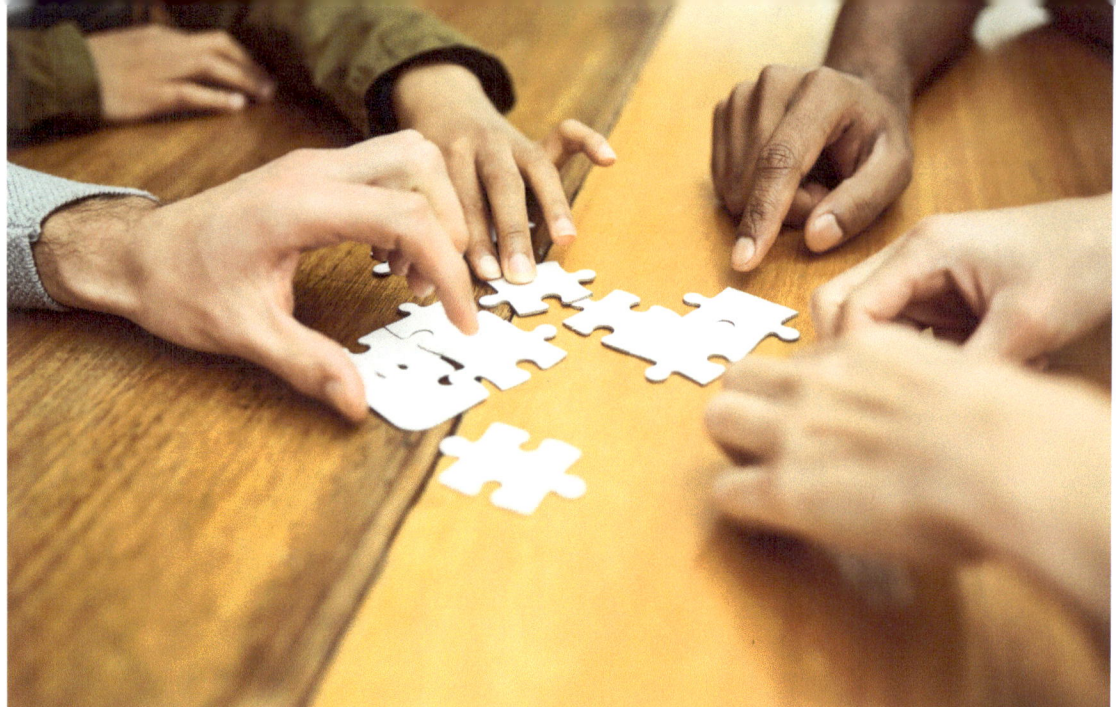

New models

While we will see some change from within, expect big tech, led especially by Amazon, to further disrupt health care. This will shift reimbursement mechanisms and drive shared risk across payers and providers. Equally significant change is emerging from China and India where the creation of identity related platforms is driving innovation at scale. At the same time, some anticipate that the reinvention of healthcare business models will come from more unexpected places.

Personalisation, data marketplaces and the application of AI are among some of the digital disruptions already impacting the provision of healthcare. A growing array of large and nimble organisations are variously seeking changes to delivery models, identifying different ways of working, reinventing HCP training and reinvigorating local, out-of-hospital care. But, many recognise that, in a way, this is just scratching the surface and believe the sector needs more fundamental change. The expectation is that this will come from disruptive new business models – either from big tech companies with access to a wealth of additional personal wellness and proxy data or from the governments looking to manage the huge population centres in the new economies of China and India.

THE NEED FOR CHANGE

Given the rising costs and population shifts, the calls for new, improved healthcare models are many and varied. But delivering the required change is no easy task. There are multiple reasons for this. Encouraging it from within is a constant battle in many organisations and systems, particularly ones which have evolved gradually or grown steadily over many years. Often the best-laid plans get bogged down in the sheer complexity of multiple legacy information systems - despite the vast sums that may have been spent on IT. Add in the challenge of encouraging lasting behaviour change and it is understandable that a sustained transition within any large entity can take years to define, test, pilot and embed. On top of this, changing culture takes much longer to adapt than installing new technology. In one 2016 UK Digital Health discussion[165] it was stated that *"clinicians and health professionals are often naturally conservative and change averse – it is often viewed as a threat to roles and responsibilities."* In South Africa it was suggested that one reason for this locally is the comparative age of GPs; many are over 50 and a good number are set in their ways – so hence they tend to push-back against digitisation. But they are also concerned that too much technology will remove them from being able to take proper care of their patients' emotional needs, *"healthcare providers are hesitant to use new technology and many GPs see the PC screen as a barrier between them and their patients."*

Whether they like it or not, established healthcare systems will however have to be ever more alert to change because, attracted by the rising levels of spend, more and more tech firms and new start-ups are lining up to get involved and maybe even take control. Whether they will, in the end, be successful is up for debate – they have tried and failed before.[166] Google started its Google Health health-records initiative in 2008, but shut it down by 2011, citing poor adoption. Microsoft's HealthVault has made similar efforts with likewise low take-up.

Perhaps the timing was wrong? Many now see that now that the widespread global availability of smartphones, with their ability to give patients access to their data whenever they want and wherever they are, has opened the door to new opportunities. Major disruptions may be coming our way. As already highlighted, new data sets that contain information about human health are hugely valuable. The more data the tech firms can handle, the more they will learn about human health, and the better the services they can offer will become.[167]

CHANGE FROM WITHIN

But don't give up on the existing players just yet. Numerous experts we talked to still believe that significant change is emerging from within the current healthcare systems - be that from governments and the systems directly or via companies in key sectors, such as pharmaceuticals and insurance. In Brussels, it was proposed that the ability of government(s) to drive collaboration across traditional silos and link health and wealth could be transformational for Western systems. Many have pointed to Singapore as leading in this area. The need, they argued, is for governments to rethink and *"support wellbeing as an investment rather than a cost."* While Western models are on most radars, there was also an alternative view which pointed to India and China as being likely centres for future data-driven healthcare innovation.

INDIAN EFFICIENCY

In Mumbai we heard that *"innovation happens when there are gaps and there are lots of gaps in India - so lots of opportunity."* Moreover, India is the only market in the world with huge price diversity – a place where you can pay $1,000 or $50,000 for the same complex procedure. Here the potential for change is tangible and we are already seeing action.[168] While previous successes of Aravind[169] and Narayana[170] in reinventing cataract and cardiac surgery for high-quality / low-cost treatment are well documented, the major future shift is very much expected to be a consequence of the way almost the entire population is now connected onto a single digital platform. In both Sydney and Singapore, as well as in Mumbai, the impact of Aadhaar[171] linking healthcare data to identity[172] was seen as highly significant. *"With over 1bn people using Aadhaar there is volume advantage in terms of available datasets"* and, as financial inclusion becomes more integrated, the opportunities for change from, for example, microfinance and health insurance are considerable.[173]

While there are several other nations making significant progress at integrating and sharing data (e.g. Iceland, Singapore and Sweden), they are operating with a maximum population of just a few million. What is happening in India, with over a billion people, will not only have huge local impact but also has the potential to set new standards globally. Although a number of concerns need to be addressed such as ensuring informed consent of those who are illiterate; managing the strict privacy regulation; and understanding the consequence of the threatened data inversion legislation (the forced repatriation of data to India), the sheer scale of what is underway in India in terms of the harmonised data sets of so many people on one platform is enormous. Many are now watching what is going on with great interest. With the high-level support of the Modi government and associated initiatives such as Digital India and Start-up India all gaining traction, confidence is clearly building. India is creating a new model for its own healthcare system that may well leap-frog many other nations. One suggestion in Mumbai was that, as it is already so intertwined into the global health care procedures from years of BPO activity, then, as India innovates, so its' advances will quickly become integrated into other systems.

CHINESE MOMENTUM

But it is not just India that could deliver wider change. Also well-worth tracking are healthcare developments in China, where some suggest that major advances in technology that are now being applied to healthcare may well have global reach. Certainly, momentum is building fast and China is making great progress in many core areas – from the adoption of robotics within surgery to the application of AI to diagnosis. Although initial emphasis for many Chinese healthcare companies is on the huge domestic market, many see that the 'Made in China for China' focus will soon shift to be global. Just as has occurred in telecoms with Huawei, other Chinese firms such as Tencent, Baidu and Alibaba are arguably now also 'shaping the global future of tech.'[174] Whether or not coming from the 'pure-play' healthcare-focused firms like iCarbonX or new health apps on broader platforms such as WeChat and Alipay, the scale of the impact on healthcare that could emerge from China is significant, particularly given a fundamentally different outlook inherent to its current healthcare model. In our Toronto discussion, it was, for example, pointed out that China has a completely different attitude to the doctor/patient relationship as *"the patient determines the efficacy of his or her treatment and so whether or not to pay the doctor. Maybe this approach could be adopted in the West?"* New models in Chinese healthcare built around a different philosophy coupled with better and large data sets are emerging from multiple directions and are rapidly being applied to hundreds of millions of patients - delivering quick proof of new concepts at scale. Coupled with already huge and fast-rising domestic venture investments, several in our workshops feel that much of healthcare in the second half of 21st century could have a distinct Chinese flavour.

NEW PHARMA MODELS

In terms of specific sectors within healthcare, there was almost universal consensus that, alongside elements of insurance, the pharmaceutical industry is ripe for disruption as a result of the growth in patient data. In London, the view was that many are already exploring how to break funding silos, while in Singapore it was suggested that *"pharmaceutical firms should only be reimbursed if their drugs work – and can prove that the targeted benefits can be delivered."* Assuming the growing demands for higher quality healthcare continue, that patients are increasingly data-aware and that all parties agree that change is needed, the UK discussions also suggested that the better use of patient data would increase the potential for multiple future shifts. These include:

- Using data focused on outcomes to change reimbursement models and drive shared risk,

- Policy and process changes with payers and providers increasingly in alignment,

- Leveraging data to bridge the silos between social care, medical devices, hospitals and chronic care,

- Integrating data to get the whole customer view as well as shared interests,

- Bringing society along as a partner for change with individuals willing to provide their data to support it,

- Developing 'consumer products that care' rather than care products for consumers, and

- Data cooperatives driving the buyers of data – that are willing to pay and understand the value of data.

In Frankfurt, many pointed out that the patient will probably become the co-producer of care in the future and that many changes in healthcare are likely to be patient-driven rather than solely powered by the corporates. A focus on, and support for, more personalised and preventative healthcare *"will also add pressure on the current "artificially high-level pricing of drugs."* Indeed, it may herald the end of the blockbuster era for pharmaceuticals. *"Progress with cancer care and type 1 diabetes may well set new precedents for a world in which improved availability of data will drive new revenue streams."*

BIG TECH MOVES

Alongside the multiple shifts from within healthcare systems, many of the big tech organisations are also making some major moves in healthcare. Learning from their past mistakes, many believe that as patients are now more used to sharing information on the cloud, this time around they will be more prepared to trust and share their sensitive health records.

Although many of the big tech companies are highly secretive about their 'special projects', it's an open secret that they are all busy hiring talent and buying or backing external health-care start-ups. With hundreds of PhDs recently moving from the public research centres within key universities into Alphabet, Amazon and Apple as well as Facebook and Microsoft, the signals are clear that healthcare-focused activities within the varied skunk works are escalating. The question is how fast they will move and with what intention. Current acquisitions and announcements already suggest major movements.

Several shifts are visible – *"look for example at Health Records embedded in the next version of Apple's Health App and the launch of (Alphabet's) Cityblock Health"* was one suggestion. Apple is indeed embedding the next generation of sensors within all its products to capture and analyse more personal health data; **Flatiron Health** (see case study) is building its capacity to turn health data into insights transforming EHR data into analysable, actionable information; Microsoft started a health-care division in Cambridge, England in September 2017 which will devise medical algorithms of its own; and Alphabet spin-out **Verily** (see case study) wants to be the R&D partner for the world's leading life sciences companies. It is looking to become "the OS for healthcare." These are all in play. Other options being speculated upon include Google, Amazon or Apple moving into the EHR space by purchasing one of the major existing EHR vendors.

In many of our discussions, the future focus for healthcare innovation is still very much seen to be around the US big tech firms where *"the sheer scale, wealth and reach are a major driver of future change."* This is particularly true of the ones with nearly global reach as part of their existing services. In Sydney, it was felt that *"by 2030, a growing number of non-traditional entrants will have enabled a more specialised consumer-centric care system."* It won't be easy to generate a change in behaviour, but, assuming the aim is profit creation, most likely from data markets, then, alongside the need to generate higher levels of consumer acceptance, the Australian view was that there may also be a few political and regulatory hurdles to negotiate. Moreover, if we get it right, there will be a greater focus on preventative healthcare with the doctor increasingly *'riding side-car.'*

AMAZON HEALTH

Across the vast majority of our events, time and time again the biggest source of disruption for the future of healthcare was seen to be coming from one organisation – **Amazon** (see case study) and its secretive lab 1492: *"Amazon has made the biggest strides so far"*.[175] It has already initiated significant change in how drugs are sold and is making shopping for healthcare easier for both customers and medical professionals.[176] It is bringing the efficiencies proven elsewhere into the healthcare supply chain. Several see that Amazon could, for instance, soon build or, more likely, acquire a health insurance platform.

In addition, for more patient data focused services, although some see that Alphabet and Apple's current investments may have greater visible impact in the short term, the often-repeated opinion in our discussions was that *"Amazon will own all your data in the end."*[177] In San Francisco, one assessment was that *"even though coming from outside the sector, Amazon could be the catalyst that creates a 'single' more unified (US) system."* Many others agreed with this. *"I have invested in 18 new healthcare ventures – 17 of them use AWS."* While that does not imply that Amazon has access to the data, the fact that it is already sitting on its servers then, should permission be granted then integration and interrogation can easily follow on. Although recent announcements around the use of employee data[178] have been assessed as Amazon's next move in healthcare, this was considered to be *"just the beginning."*

Another suggestion was that *"EPIC had its time but failed to take advantage of the opportunity,"* so *"Amazon will take the lead and may run the whole marketplace."* This *"may well be the monetization platform for health data in the US (and beyond). It has the capability, the reach and the intent."* The view, again in San Francisco, was unequivocal – *"Just look at the signs. It is happening: It is the same as Einstein in Salesforce*[179] *- one organisation will be able to integrate all the data and in healthcare that company will be Amazon."* Some also asked whether *"we may all see the end of our social security number as how our identity is managed changes."*

There seems to be a belief in the impact of Amazon, not just because of its wealth and reach, but also because of its proven approach to business model innovation. As mentioned in the accompanying case study, it has consistently demonstrated the capability to deliver highly efficient reinventions of existing systems and to do that with world-leading levels of customer service and satisfaction.

Benefits for the Patient

The common core ambitions for many of the new models that are evolving are two-fold: Maximising system efficiency and vastly improving customer satisfaction. Whether from outside or inside healthcare, from India, China, Europe or the US, these innovations should improve patients' lives. Greater convenience, lower costs, faster service, better engagement, smoother processes and enhanced personal health are all central.

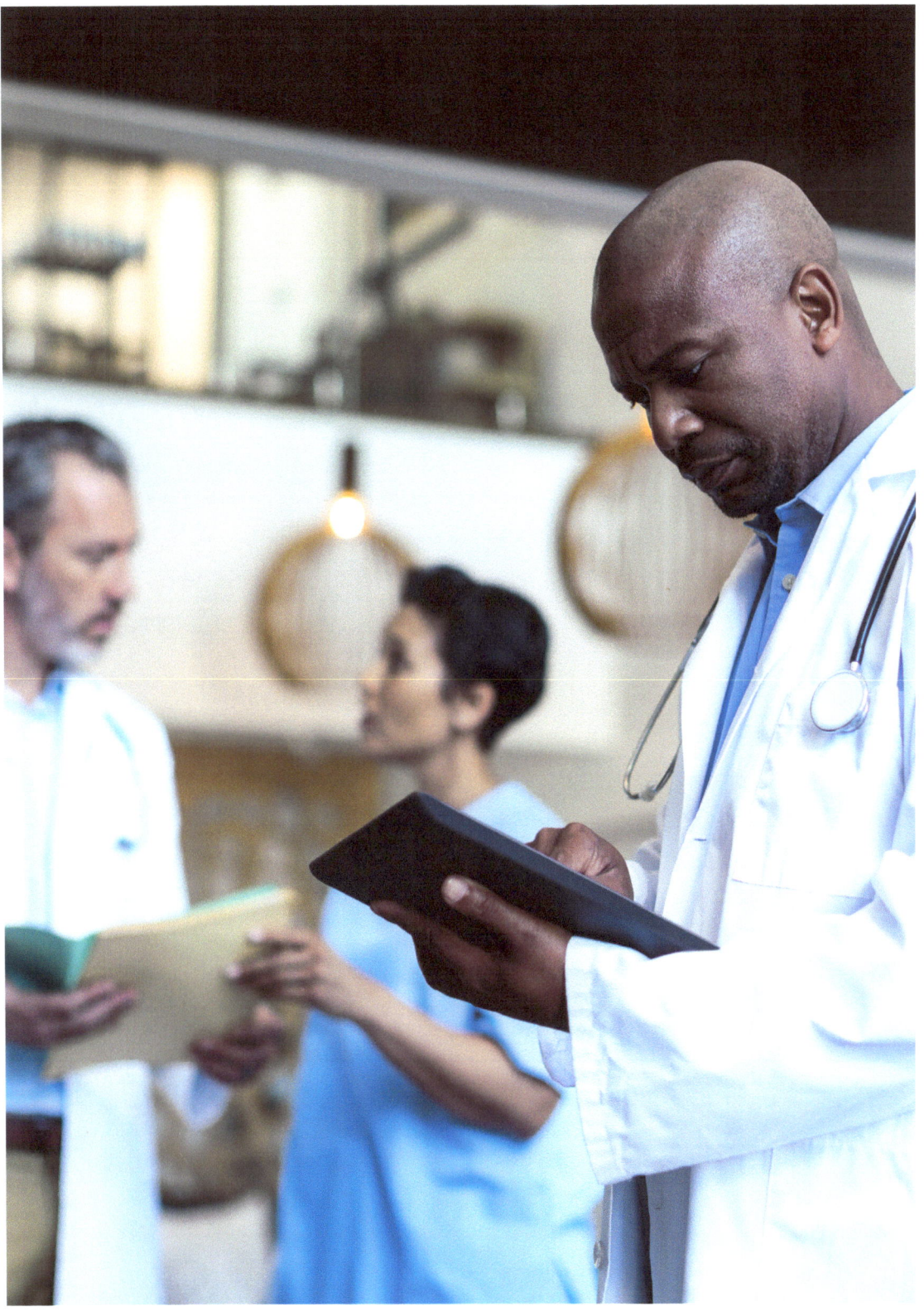

CASE STUDY:

verily

Officially launched in 2015, Verily is a subsidiary of Alphabet focused on life sciences and healthcare. A spin-out of the Google X lab, the company's mission is "to make the world's health data useful so that people enjoy longer and healthier lives." Verily develops tools and devices to collect, organize and activate health data, and creates interventions to prevent and manage disease.[180]

It is creating tools and platforms to enable more continuous health data collection for timely decision-making, running longitudinal studies to better understand ways to predict and prevent disease onset and undertaking significant joint efforts with partners to 'radically transform' the way healthcare is delivered.

Indeed, most projects are in partnership with established major healthcare companies where Verily can bring its advanced hardware, software and scientific data skills to bear – collaborating is fundamental to the approach as the company applies its expertise, learns and, in doing so, builds up access to a wealth of health data. It wants to be the R&D partner for the world's leading life sciences companies.[181]

Key areas of focus to date include developing sensors, such as miniaturized continuous glucose monitors for people with diabetes, analysis of physiological and environmental data linked to clinical studies, improving surgical robotics, developing machine-learning driven retinal imaging solutions; and developing tools to better analyse and report performance data across healthcare systems.[182]

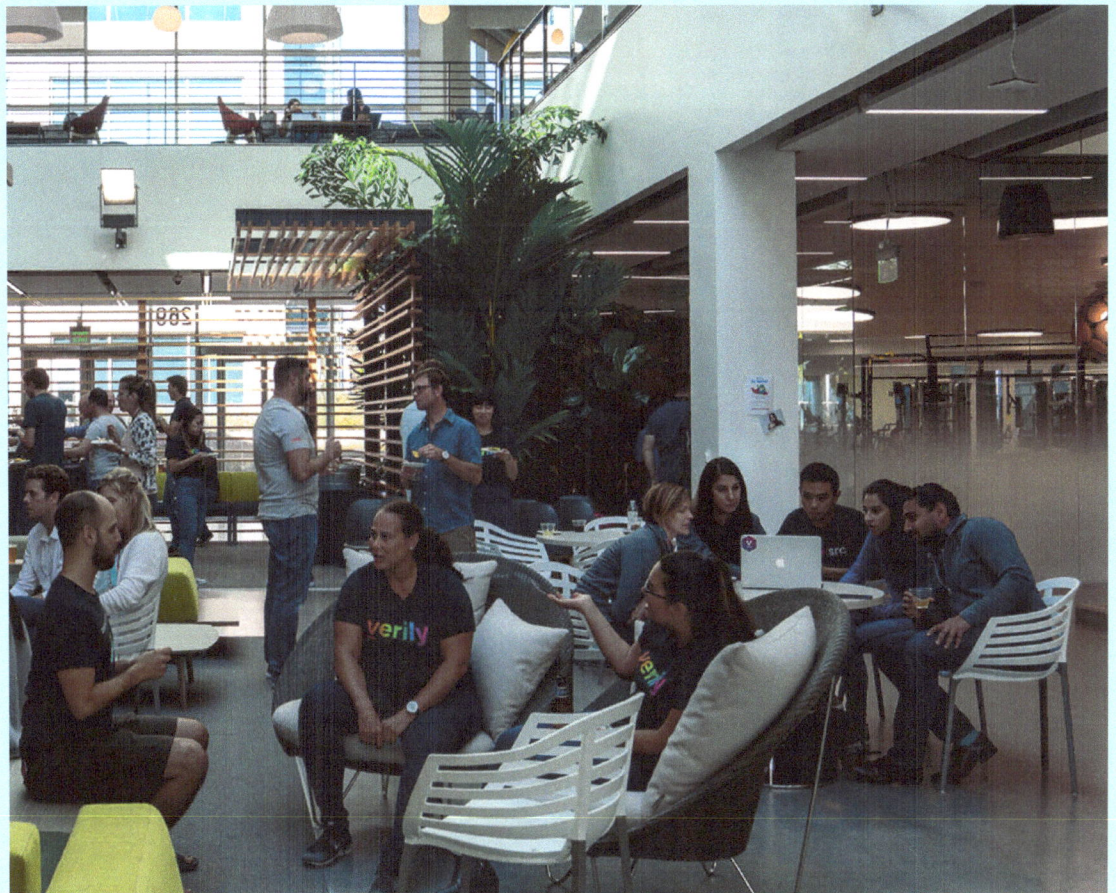

Presently, Verily makes around $1bn of revenue from research grants and development fees from its collaborators.[183] Assumptions about future plans include the idea that it will sell access to its healthcare platform, disease data and software to the broader health sector.[184] Others see that Verily could become the OS for all healthcare devices.[185] In January 2018, Dr Jessica Mega, Verily's Chief Medical Officer, suggested that it is "Google Maps for health."[186] Clearly there are many options ahead, but as one of the Alphabet's major 'Other Bets' expectations of future impact are high.

CASE STUDY:

amazon

Few would doubt Amazon's ambitions in healthcare. Over recent years, it has made significant investments, recruited leading-edge talent, made some initial announcements and is seen as the biggest disruptive threat by many leaders across the health sector. The question is not whether Amazon Health will be big, but rather just how big?

Some already see the ability to apply many of its existing capabilities to the sector. For example:[187]

- **Comprehensive customer records** - providing 'complete longitudinal information and intelligent analytics at every point of care' that integrates all patient data - health, clinical and personal.

- **Personalized content and user experience** - having intelligible information and recommendations based on a full view of a patient's health history, condition and provider interactions with feedback / advice.

- **Price transparency and choice** – giving the world's first 'comprehensive view of cost options for treatments or medications' supported with intelligent assistance in choosing between them.

- **Quality reviews** - a 'single source for trustworthy quality ratings of hospitals, physicians and other health care providers' that sets new standards and validates its accuracy.

Other organisations are focused on achieving one of these, but as some argue, Amazon already does them all to an exemplary standard and just needs to apply them to healthcare. In addition, it does this with one of the highest rated customer satisfaction globally – many times better than the norm for healthcare. As with many of its previous new platforms, many see the recently announced partnership between Amazon, Berkshire Hathaway and J.P. Morgan as the opportunity to experiment internally on 1.2m employees and get this all working very well before expanding to the wider population.

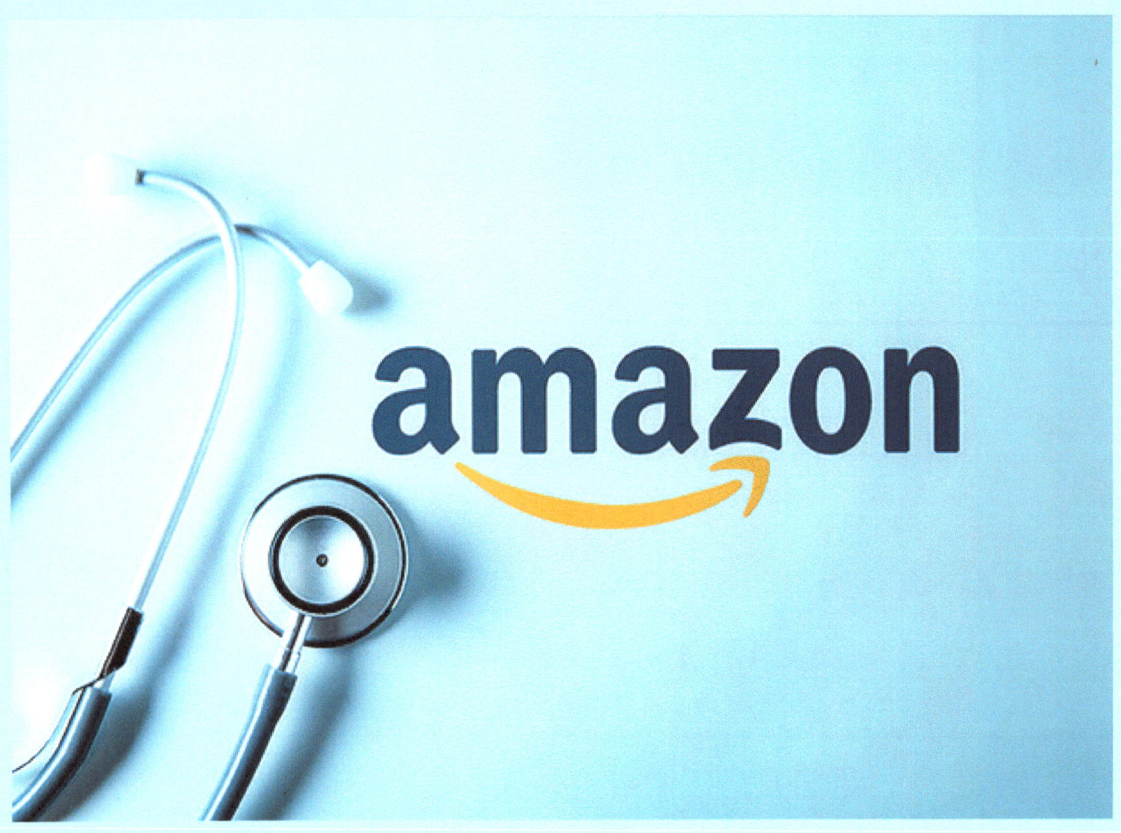

Beyond this, others have suggested[188] the potential in applying Amazon Prime and Amazon Flex quality and reliability of delivery to healthcare products, using the Whole Foods footprint as a base for health services like those provided by CVS MinuteClinic, integrating the passive data capture seen in Amazon Go stores to hospitals to improve efficiency, and using its considerable data analytics capabilities to integrate patient records. Others expect another go at disrupting the pharmacy sector, a potential $50bn Amazon opportunity in the US alone.[189]

However, looking further, additional opportunities include integrating Alexa insights on individual behaviours from within the home into personalised health data profiles, as well as applying analytics to much of the millions of terabytes of health-related data already on the Amazon cloud service, AWS, that some see as potentially accounting for 50% of Amazon's future revenues. Add on more AI innovations and new technology emerging from the 3000 plus R&D experts in the company's lab 1492[190] and the potential is significant and growing.

Like other potential disruptors, Amazon clearly sees the 17% of US GDP spent on healthcare as a highly attractive opportunity to provide new platforms that can improve efficiency and reduce cost. Unlike many others, it has most of the ingredients to hand, plus deep pockets to fund necessary add-on acquisitions and buy talent, deepening relationships with the 64% of US households that have Amazon Prime and over 300m existing customers worldwide.[191] Expect a steady stream of revelations of new means of making more of health data over the next few years - and the corresponding drop in incumbent companies shares with each announcement.[192]

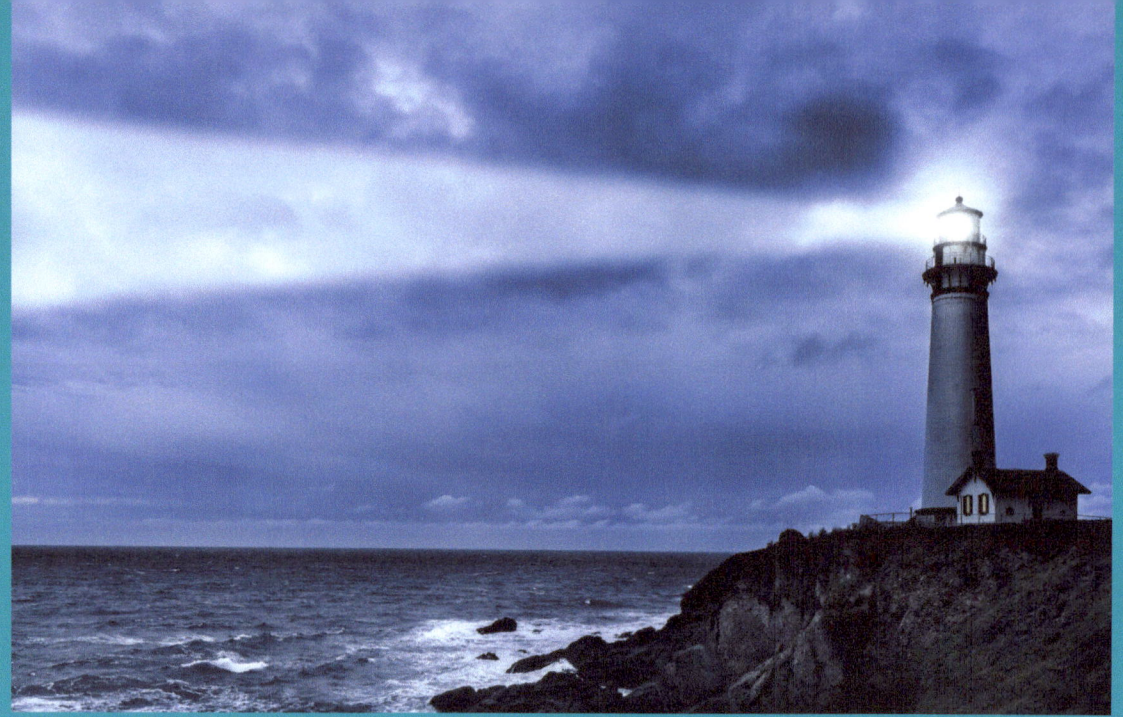

Emerging issues

Lastly, across our discussions we can see several issues that are fast emerging on to the radar. While not yet equally visible, nor having the same significance, in every location, there are nevertheless topics over which there is increasingly hot debate. They are issues where there is yet to be clear consensus on the challenge and some may have very different political and commercial implications in the future. They are however also topics that could have manifest impact on how the future of patient data actually plays out, how and where greatest benefit can be achieved and who may gain the most. These are matters about which many organisations well need to both understand the core drivers and develop a firm point of view on so that, as we move forward, collaboration can occur between the key parties – those who can deliver the ambitions around a more patient centric approach to healthcare and its intrinsic use of data.

These four areas are:

Data Sovereignty – More nations seek to restrict the sharing of health data beyond their borders. This is driven by concerns around national security, the desire to protect commercial interest and the different cultural attitudes to privacy. Consequently, there is a corresponding push-back against some global ambitions with India and China potentially gaining the upper hand.

Digital Inequality – As advances roll out, there is growing concern around those who are not included in the "system". Several hope that, with more and better data, health inequality can be reduced but others see a widening divide between those with access to technology and those without. Adapting to change is a real challenge for healthcare workers and patients alike. To help drive progress, many want outcome-based measures to be standardised, but many regulators are behind the curve. How countries deal with these is as much political and commercial as it is technological.

Privatisation of Health Information - The privatisation of medical knowledge and the increased use of new 'secret software' challenges the potential for healthcare data to be more open source or, at least, shared within an agreed governance system.

The Value of Health Data – It is clear that patient data can be used to drive both social and economic benefit. As public understanding grows so will consensus about its worth. As this shift happens, those who can best grasp its multiple roles in, and value to, society, and render these things comprehensible to others, will likely have the more powerful voice.

Each are explored in the following pages.

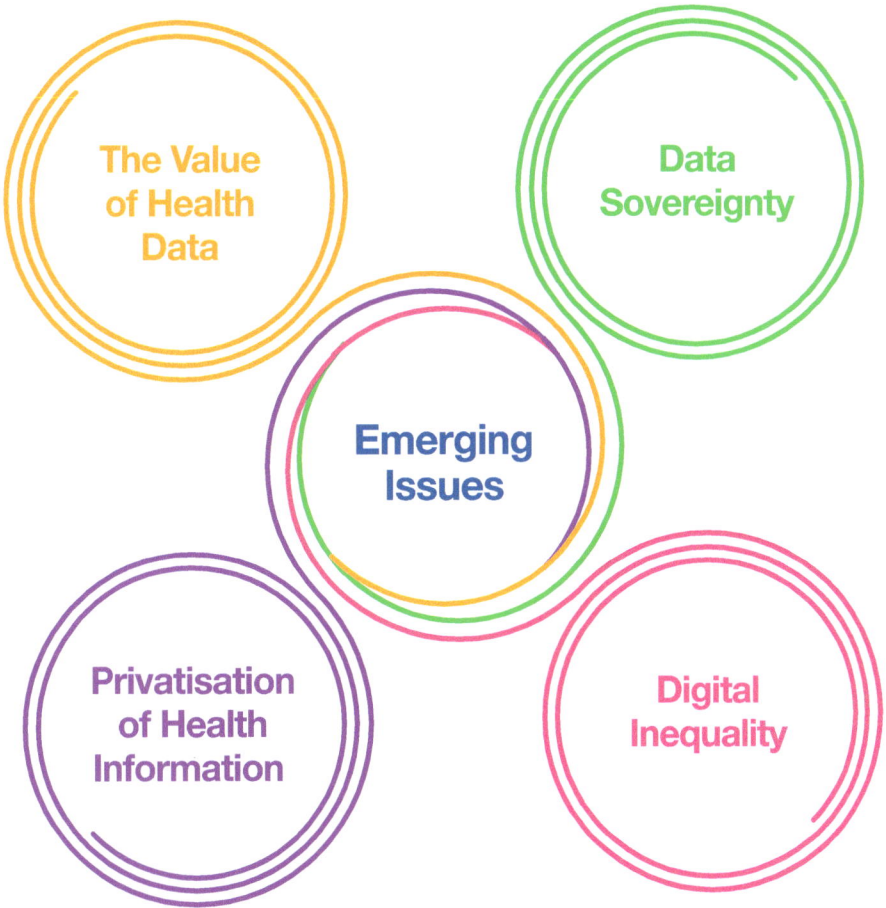

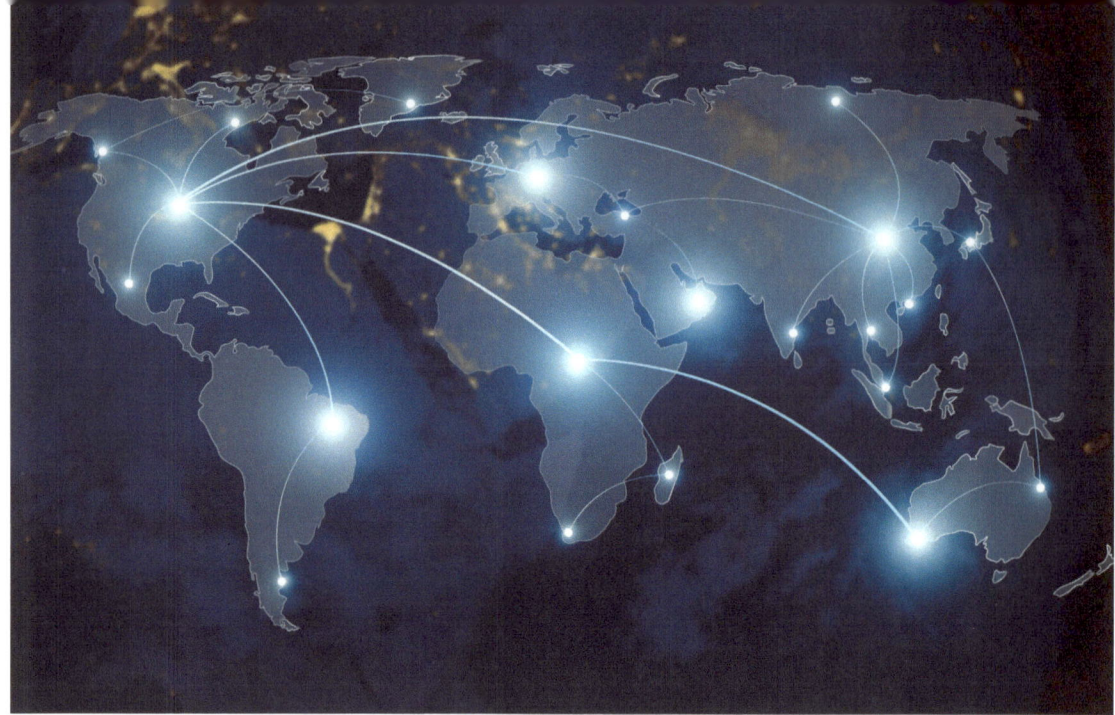

Data sovereignty

More nations seek to restrict the sharing of health data beyond their borders. This is driven by concerns around national security, the desire to protect commercial interest and the different cultural attitudes to privacy. Consequently, there is a corresponding push-back against some global ambitions with India and China potentially gaining the upper hand.

Data sovereignty refers to the fact that data in a cloud service provider may well be subject to the jurisdiction of more than one country.[193] This has specific implications for the health sector. As more organisations seek to integrate multiple patient data sources from around the world, accommodating local and regional rules is a growing concern. In parallel, as more data moves to the cloud, traditional geopolitical boundaries are being challenged and questions are increasingly being raised about where exactly it is being stored, and under what jurisdictions it lies.

From a health research perspective many believe that access to global databases could have the potential to transform real-world evidence in medicine and healthcare. For example, terabytes of unstructured data from many different, real-world data sources ranging from EMRs, genetic profiles, phenotypic data and mHealth devices could be explored in order to find unexpected patterns and identify possible new solutions. Genetic data in particular can provide deeper insights into the nature and size of the sub-population groups who could be served by new treatments. Many new healthcare innovators, from Alphabet and Amazon to DigiMe and iCarbonX, are keen to exploit this global data opportunity. By definition they all assume they will operate in multiple markets. However, this is not a given. As one expert noted *"the internationalisation of data is not guaranteed."* To be effective in the future organisations should be cognisant of, and sensitive to, the sovereign requirements of other countries. In a world of rising nationalism and increasing scepticism about the benefits of globalisation, much of which is negatively associated with companies based on the west coast of the US, this is no easy task.

Although open to the benefits of big data sharing in healthcare, many experts are also cautious about its implications and agree that in many regions *"we will increasingly have to consider the issue of data sovereignty."* Certainly, several governments are deploying a variety of discourses, policies and practices in order to constrain what many wish to be global to the local level. More nation states are claiming sovereignty over both the technological architecture that enables transnational information flows, and the communications themselves. Academic literature and public policy refer to these claims of *"supreme authority"* over ICT and its content respectively as technological sovereignty and information sovereignty. These can often overlap since the differences between them are not clear-cut.[194]

In its 2018 Tech Trends report, Deloitte highlights data sovereignty as a key issue for the future and suggest why different regions are taking alternative views.[195] "In Northern Europe historical context related to civil liberties, privacy, and nation-state data collection may make the topic of data sovereignty particularly sensitive and highly politicized. Across the Americas, Europe, and Asia Pacific, active discussions are under way between the government and private sectors to shape regulation. In all corners of the world - including South Africa, Italy, Brazil, and China - public providers are racing to build 'national' clouds in advance of evolving privacy laws. Region-specific timeframes and barriers reflect these considerations, indicating either the expected window for investments and policies to mature or a cautious buffer due to the complexities involved."

Data sovereignty is generally allied to the principle that data stored in a country is subject to its laws and regulations. In Europe an additional layer of protection is added because the private data of citizens falls under the sovereignty of the EU as well as that of sovereignty of their individual nations. With its wide mandate, the European GDPR legislation, covering all EU data irrespective of location, is also setting a new benchmark for non-EU jurisdictions. This is particularly the case for several US based companies as, in the main, much European personal data is currently processed by US service providers such as Cisco, Google, Facebook and Microsoft. Some data sovereignty regulations, for instance Russia's 2015 On Personal Data (OPD) law, go even further and not only specify who has power over data but also mandates that any data pertaining to a country's citizens must physically reside in that country.

Throughout our conversations it became clear that geography and national identity are becoming of increasing significance when considering the sharing of data. In some areas, such as Singapore, the primary issue was around security and how to protect its citizens if personal data was housed outside the state. Indeed, Singapore offered perhaps our most extreme view in favour of maximising data sovereignty by arguing the case for limiting data sharing on the basis of national security: *"Our existing laws restrict the sharing of personal data (including health data) beyond the national boundary"* plus there is a potential risk that *"future warfare may use health data"* and as *"no-one has yet worked out the extent to which patient data can compromise government security"* so it cannot be shared.

By contrast, in South Africa data sovereignty was more a concern around "the risk of commercial exploitation." Here, the government has restricted the sharing of blood samples with US based

101

companies for genetic profiling. The worry is that 'cheap' African data can be used as a valuable reference set that can then be exploited commercially. It was suggested that one reason for this may well be due to the US laws around privacy and genetic regulation. In Sydney, as a follow-on comment, it was observed "US privacy legislation only protects US residents' data and not that from other countries' citizens."

Elsewhere the argument for greater data sovereignty falls between these extremes but it is perhaps in India where the most significant actions are now having impact. There, the planned legislation around the use of personal data (best summarised in the India Stack[196] proposal - the ambitious and controversial project of creating a unified software platform to bring India's population into the digital age) sees the significant repatriation of Indian citizens' data taking effect in the next few years. This is similar to the Russian OPD legislation and current practice in China. If this goes ahead as expected, India may well also restrict personal data sharing to within its national boundaries, where it can then be managed and, as best suits, monetised by Indian, and not foreign, companies. The same principles will apply to financial and health data. In Europe questions around sovereignty are intrinsically tied up with the those around privacy. In the US, however, experts were more confident that this could be addressed and therefore supportive of the benefits of openly sharing health data globally.

Concern was specifically expressed in the UK which has the world's largest publicly funded health service and, as such, one of the most comprehensive health datasets. Its patient records are, maybe, uniquely suited for driving the development of powerful algorithms and, so, several felt they should be protected from commercial exploitation. *"What you don't want is somebody using NHS data as a learning set for the next generation of algorithms and then moving the algorithm to San Francisco and selling it, so all the profits come back to another jurisdiction."* To go some way to addressing this, NHS Digital has begun to provide guidance on how care providers can best choose offshore public cloud services to store patient data.[197]

Some have also argued for a more equal geographic distribution of the value extracted from data. Currently, most big data refineries are based in America, or are controlled by US firms, and it is through them that a significant amount of innovation takes place. As the data economy progresses in other markets this may not continue. Europe has, for instance, proposed a digital tax. Others disagree. Some in our San Francisco discussion suggested that the fact that patients will increasingly own their own data is a major driver against greater data sovereignty. *"They, and not federal government can choose what happens to their data."* One view was *"this sounds a bit Big Brother and could limit cross country sharing and movement of data."* Moreover *"it seems as though other countries are using data sovereignty as an excuse for not making progress"* and *"we have bigger issues to address."* In addition, *"worrying about this is like moving the deckchairs on the Titanic – legislation is 5 years behind what is already happening."* The feeling was that while other countries may be concerned about data sovereignty, *"in the US we are moving ahead and are more focused on making better use of our healthcare information."*

Given the strong and varied views on this pivotal topic, it is clear that the ambitions for international companies to act as conduits for multinational, or even global, shifts towards more patient control may well need to be modified within more localised priorities. As trust between nations becomes increasingly challenged and fears of cyber-attacks are on the rise, perhaps it is unsurprising that data sovereignty has become a priority for some. Should the protectionist approach become more widely adopted it may well give highly populated countries such as India and China an advantage when it comes to medical research. Both countries have populations of over 1.2 billion, increasingly connected people. Access to their data will provide a wealth of information and understanding. Those in smaller markets may find it hard to challenge.

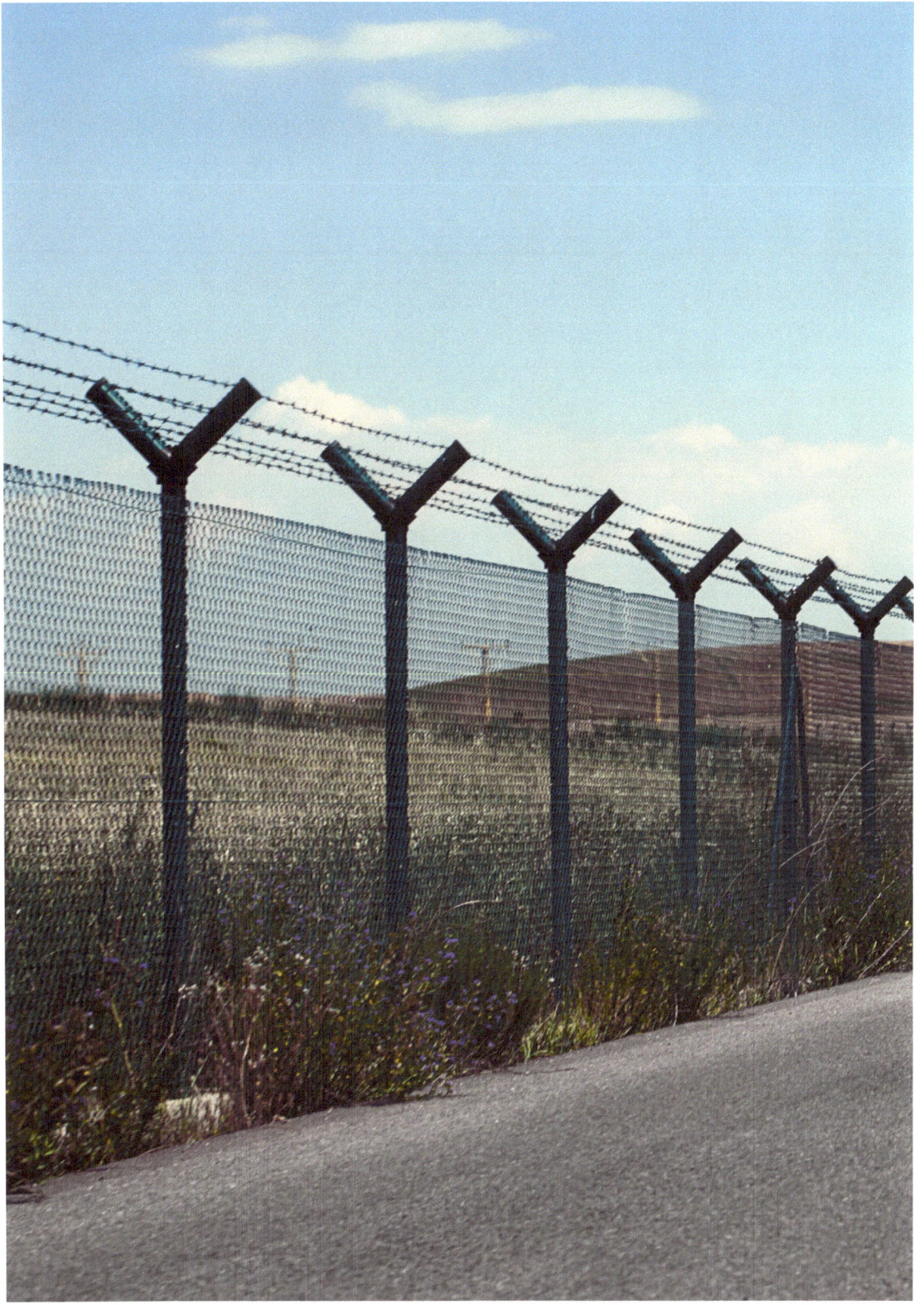

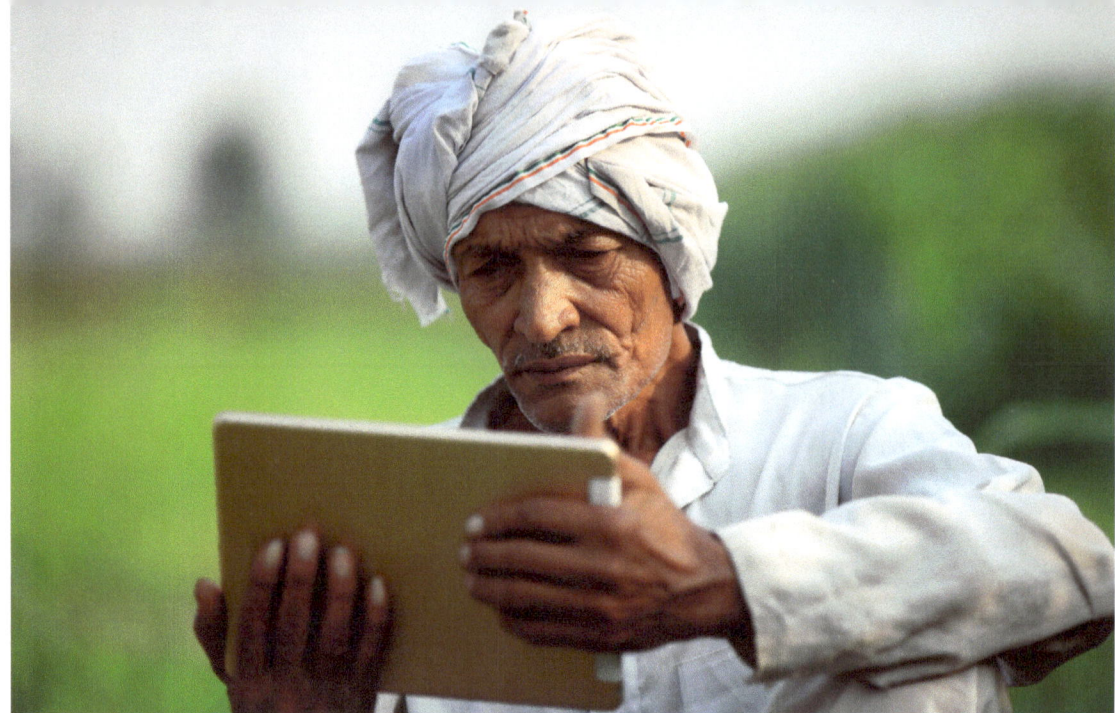

Digital inequality

As advances roll out, there is growing concern around those who are not included in the "system". Several hope that, with more and better data, health inequality can be reduced but others see a widening divide between those with access to technology and those without. Adapting to change is a real challenge for healthcare workers and patients alike. To help drive progress, many want outcome-based measures to be standardised, but many regulators are behind the curve. How countries deal with these is as much political and commercial as it is technological.

While greater use of more and better patient data is the global ambition for everyone, there are several issues which may well constrain adoption and impact. Although the ideal is that the better and more efficient use of patient data will benefit everyone, some indications suggest, in the next decade at least, its impact may well only benefit the few. Across all of our discussions, there were three key areas of concern – access, skills and standards.

ACCESS INEQUALITY

Globally, there is great hope that a more digital approach to healthcare will both increase efficiency and increase access. Given that nearly 70% of the global population still does not yet receive decent healthcare, there is a strong belief that data-driven technology has the potential to transform the situation. The question is how much? Telemedicine is already having significant impact and seeding wider change. Across Africa and Asia, the addition of more intelligent systems is expected to further improve remote access. At the same time, while the focus is often on developing economies, there may be just as many challenges in improving access in the 'developed' world.

The risk of a widening healthcare divide was highlighted as a major concern was in several locations.[198] Take South Africa for example. It has one of most advanced private healthcare systems on the continent and yet many believe that the public health service is unfit for purpose with a doctor-patient ratio of 0.8 per 1,000, lower than Brazil, Russia, India and China. In Johannesburg the view was that *"ineffective government support and inadequate investment in the public sector means that the majority will remain without access to health data that is only available through private healthcare systems."* Priority investment by the private sector and poor management from government result in some feeling that that access to new technologies and services for the masses may well be 5 to 10 years behind the leaders. Elsewhere, others added that for many *"economic and social challenges are leading to more inequality of outcomes."*[199] Participants in Dubai also recognised the challenge of extending healthcare reach beyond the private sector seeing that *"we have lots of new technology solutions which are designed to improve patient care, but many are in their infancy. They are not reaching those who most need them, and the cost of supply is a major issue."*

Another view was that many developing countries have less data silos than in Europe and the US and so, as with mobile payments a decade ago, they have the opportunity to leap-frog legacy systems. The rising penetration of smartphones is having particular impact as shown in the graph below. Several see that developing countries will *"go mobile first and challenge existing models."* Clearly issues around literacy and numeracy add an additional layer of complexity but in India there was great optimism that healthcare is on the cusp of change. Again, much hope is being placed on India's centralised data system, Aadhaar. In London, it was proposed that *"Africa can teach the West a lot about health care"* as mobile data access in key groups (e.g. refugees, migrants etc.) has been shown to deliver significant benefit: *"Mobile platforms will increase accessibility."*

Richer economies also have challenges. An important early US-focused insight was that *"while many health apps are used by the healthy and the worried well, reaching the 5% of patients that incur 50% of healthcare costs remains a major challenge: Comorbidity will continue to drive the greatest spend."* In Sydney, it was suggested that there is no lack of data on the 5% with comorbidity who suffer from multiple conditions today. The question going forward is whether more information will enable us to take better care of them or indeed enable patients to take more care of themselves? If the answer is no, should we consider a different approach? As highlighted in the map below, there are many countries where there are a large number of adults with three of more chronic conditions which drive compound impact – both on the ability to treat and the costs of doing so. While the US has over a third of its adult population in this category, across many OECD nations the average is 1 in 5. As a response to this, in Brussels it was suggested that *"maybe we need to change the narrative around digital health and provide more incentives to use technology at key points"* – with the ambition of *"better managing (and preventing) the transition from healthy to ill."*

DRUG PRICING

Several experts see that more transparent data across healthcare could have a major impact on pricing and therefore access to important drugs. If we can all see the price of drugs in different markets, will the advent of 'international prescriptions' make purchasing easier – and what role will technology companies like Amazon (again) play here? What happens when there is total transparency of cost to the patient and they can choose to buy from anywhere?

Moreover, given that over-prescription, especially of antibiotics, is such a problem today, if healthcare is rewarded more on outcomes, as is the case in some instances in China, will doctors and providers including pharma be paid when their treatment works but not when it does not? *"If only 40% of cancer drugs work – why charge if they don't bring benefit? How can this be arbitrated? Will greater transparency of impact (and so reimbursement) change GP prescription behaviours?"*

AGEING

A specific focus in Boston was on how to give more support to the ageing population and enhance care in the home. There is a *"growing 'isolation epidemic' of people living on their own with no social infrastructure and little understanding of technology."* Maybe *"over the next decade this will change with the wide-scale adoption of more monitoring, more in-home sensing and a broader range of technology enabled human support. As a result, the care-giver will be able to better understand the healthcare needs of a patient before they even walk into the room."* Greater understanding of an individual's health and lifestyle gleaned through regular monitoring and data collection at home will provide context and richness that in theory should allow more focused treatment. In addition, *"there will be greater transparency of needs, a rise in care coordination and navigation and more care delivered in the home than in medical sites."* Key enablers here include *"information integration between community and medical providers, a rise in co-living and co-habitation, better resource reallocation and more risk-sharing."*

No one expects technology to deliver the solution to what is the cultural problem around how richer societies in particular treat the old. That said, many felt at least it could in some way assist by relieving some of the difficulties of isolated living.

Older Adults With Three Or More Chronic Conditions

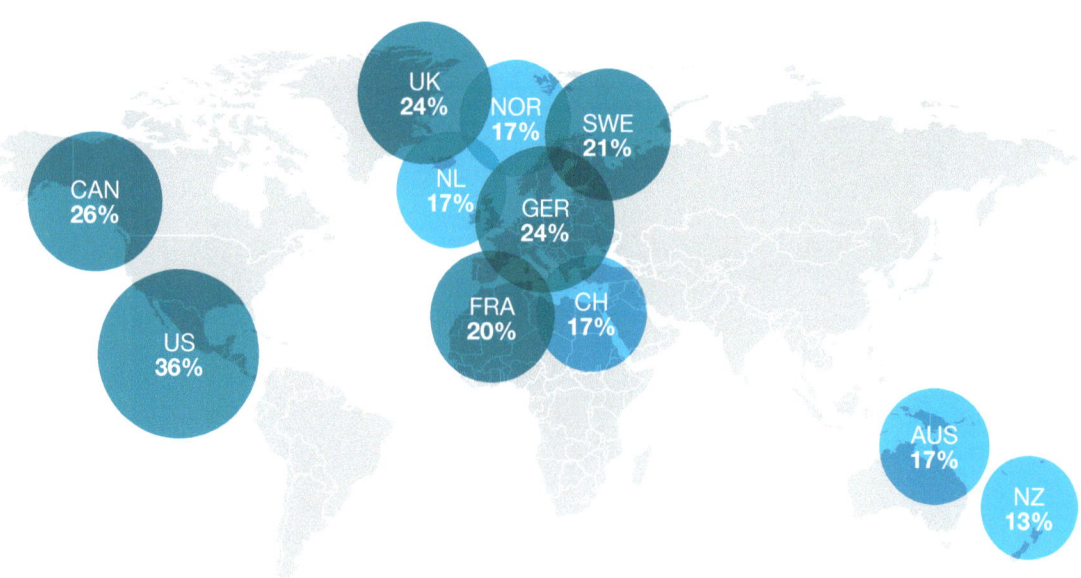

Source: 2017 Commonwealth Fund International Health Policy Survey of Older Adults

LITERACY AND UNDERSTANDING

However, underpinning much of the potential benefits of increased use of data in the delivery of healthcare are other concerns about the level of public understanding of health issues and how best to communicate in order to influence positive behaviour. For example, some in our workshops wondered how literate you need to be to understand how to manage your health? In Oslo, the question was raised as to whether *"the typical citizen understands the concept of probability"*, while in San Francisco it was highlighted that the average US citizen has a reading level of grade 5 or 6. Indeed, over 20% of Americans are *'not able to locate information in text'* or *'integrate easily identifiable pieces of information'* and only 7 in 10 read books.[200] A core request therefore is how best to communicate with patients and how much information should be shared so that they can reasonably be expected to make choices. Some wondered what should be filtered. Everyone agreed that if patients are going to be given more access to their own health data, we still need to work out who is going to explain what it actually means.

DIGITAL SKILLS

The ability to understand and communicate the meaning of large amounts of data is just one of the skills needed in the future provision of healthcare. As our discussions revealed there are several emerging areas of concern. Many expect the way doctors and other healthcare professionals care for their patients will change over the next decade. There will be *"job transformation in every aspect of healthcare. In the future, there will be fewer higher paid clinicians per capita but maybe more nurse practitioners. There will be clearer standards for care and better training programs for care givers."* As more information is made available to augment individual knowledge, some propose that doctors will become more focused on the softer skills, caring for the psychological effects of illness rather than the disease itself. Others consider that healthcare will become even more business focused – one hospital manager highlighted that *"we are increasingly recruiting business analysts rather than tech expertise as the skills we need are in joining together issues and looking at workflows."*

This could all significantly impact the amount and type of training required. Diagnostics for example is a major area for tech innovation especially in countries such as India where there's just one doctor for every 1,700 people. In specialist care, that gets even more compounded. Cloud based analytics is one way around the problem and companies like Tricog are making a real difference in this area. The company uses advances in computer science, communication, algorithms, and the cloud to amplify the work of specialists. In the US neurosurgeons are already talking about halving the time to qualify by focusing earlier on key specialisms. *"How many fully trained (over trained?) HCPs do we actually need? If we can work that out, then we can significant lower the cost of health care"* was an opinion in Dubai. *"In Ethiopia healthcare officers can undertake surgery after only 4 years of training."* As appendicitis is such a leading cause of death in some parts of Africa, having someone able to perform just an appendix operation (and nothing else) could have considerable impact. So, does more personalized medicine mean more specialized doctors? In India, Narayana Healthcare surgeons perform hundreds of cardiac surgery operations each week (compared to tens in many facilities in the West) and so they can specialize within cardiac surgery to a greater degree – focusing on performing multiple identical operations.

From the discussions around AI, the short-term view is very much about augmentation and clinical decision support but, in the longer-term, jobs may well be replaced. This may be very dependent on geography: In South Africa, where there is a huge scarcity of trained doctors, the view was that *"AI would not replace the GP rather it will support them."* In San Francisco it was pointed out that *"AI will have a role to play in helping to overcome physical burnout of clinicians – and much of this burnout is currently coming from excessive documentation."* In Boston, one point was there will be an ongoing shortage of care-givers so can AI help to upskill them?

Long-term there is concern about what happens when machines are more effective than humans in fields such as radiology, pathology, pharmacy and even oncology. In Frankfurt, it was suggested that *"there is a risk that doctors will become too dependent on AI and will lose necessary skills to act without the robot – an unlearning of basic physician's skills."* There was also expectation around the potential of AI to "augment the process of hiring and training people, as it will create a supportive 'infrastructure' providing on-demand, on-time training and support.

Despite this optimism, many expressed concerns about how medical education is falling behind medical technology. In Oslo, it was pointed out that students are still being trained to hand-write prescriptions (or recipes) even though the system has gone digital – so there is already a disconnect. In addition, it was felt by some that *"doctors are not being asked to be part of IT projects – they are not invited and are also too busy keeping up with the day-to-day to be able to spare much bandwidth"* as such, in some key areas a digital skills gap is building up. In Brussels, a view was that *"digital literacy is an ongoing problem and currently the curriculum does not accommodate data understanding."* This skills gap may well delay the adoption of new approaches. As such, as was agreed in several locations, *"re-skilling and up-skilling may become a priority focus for many systems."* Healthcare professionals need to have a willingness to *"learn, unlearn and relearn"*. Ultimately most agreed that the problem is short term, *"the next generation will be more technically literate"*.

In Boston, significant change is expected as the US caregiver to senior ratio seeks to change from 1:7 (now) to 1:3 over next 20 years. There will be new innovation opportunities and business models. Similarly, *"the US crisis may be eased when job roles are separated out more cleanly so that CNAs (Certified Nursing Assistants) are supplemented by lower skill substitutes."* Here 'social prescribing' is also expected to become more prevalent, with medical providers being able to prescribe and then deliver non-medical interventions. However, maybe, as shown by the 'community coach' model,[201] the most valuable role for care workers will be how to deliver behaviour change.

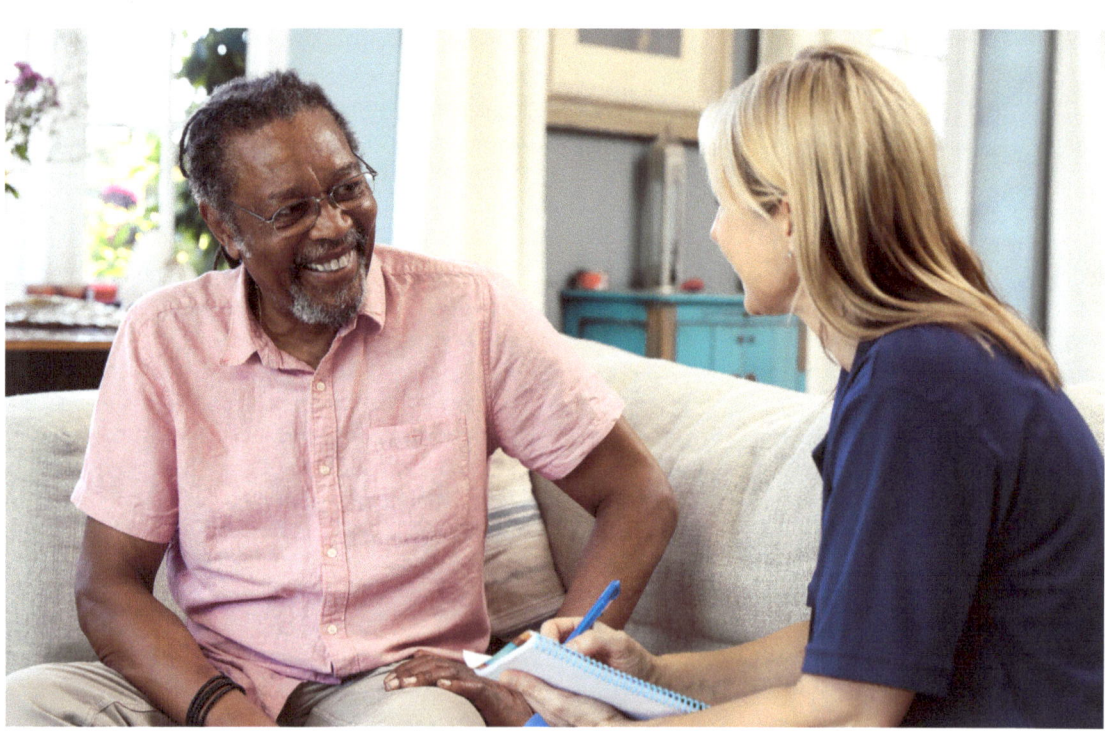

AGREED STANDARDS

As one means to help bridge the gaps, many highlight the role of digital standards. There is universal agreement that effective multi-sector and ideally multi-national (if not global) standards are a key requirement for the changes taking place around the use of patient data to have lasting impact. Public concerns around the unregulated use of data are growing and, unless controlled successfully, fears concerning how personal data is gathered, stored used and shared will become more pointed. Within this, the two primary areas of focus have been the need for standard measures and the importance of informed consent.

Improved, shared standards to measure health outcomes are believed to be a fundamental need in all locations. In part, this is driven by the predicted shift from payment for intervention (e.g. pills and the 'Rx based revenue model' for pharmaceutical firms) to payment-on-results: *"The healthcare market is evolving from a utilization marketplace to an impact marketplace."* Funders, providers, insurers, regulators and data platforms all agree that as momentum grows so does the need for standardisation of health outcomes. *"We will have to work out a new normal."*[202] Agreeing both what this should be as well as some broader digital standards, is, however, not easy. There are major commercial implications that may impact future business models.

The rapid adoption of new technologies has meant that current regulation is fragmented so needs to be consolidated and, as far as possible, future-proofed. Many agree on the requirement for a convening body to show leadership either on a regional basis (e.g. the EC) or from a global perspective (e.g. WHO). However, there are fundamental differences between European and US regulation on issues such as privacy, data protection and citizen's data rights. Most consider that regulators, almost across the board, have reached a bit of a stalemate. To address this, one suggestion was to encourage self-regulation using different industry bodies to gain consensus and then seek alignment across the sector. Singapore is already taking action but, while the models that are being adopted are proactive and ambitious, many felt it was unlikely that they will be accepted as a global standard.

Some advocate a cross-sector body which includes wellness in addition to sick care in its remit. Others fear that too much regulation early on could inhibit innovation – after all, look what happened to driverless cars. It will be slow work. In a 2016 UK discussion, it was acknowledged that *"legislators and funders of healthcare tend to be risk averse, there is a regulatory desire for certainty with a continuous concern about unintended consequences of change."* In South Africa, the Protection of Personal Information (POPI or POPIA) regulations were highlighted.[203] *"Anyone who processes health information has been invited to comment on whether the regulator should prescribe rules and what those rules should be."* In Germany, the view was that "we need networks, vocabulary and common standards to make sharing possible: We need open standards." Toronto added the requirement for *"greater evidence-based guidelines tied to clear outcomes."*

INFORMED CONSENT

Given the complex data flows, clearly articulating what is meant by informed consent is also challenging – so some see that an alternative is needed: An accountability governance model incorporating ethics and respectful data use is considered by some as a compelling substitute or complement. In Mumbai, the view was that *"if we make the end-user the custodian of data, there may be a trip wire in place."* But a key question is the extent to which poorly-educated, or extremely ill people, will really be able to understand what they are being asked to permit? The India Stack proposals[204] include at their heart a consent layer *"which allows data to move freely and securely to democratize the market for data."* Concerns were raised that, with over 1.2bn Indians coming into this framework, there will be a significant number who may not be aware what they are giving consent to.

This topic was also explored in depth in Sydney. *"The current consent system does not work given the growing predominance of technology. The existing regulation is not fit for purpose."* In addition, *"in Australia the current privacy act[205] and state legislation is very fragmented."* Moreover *"there is little consumer understanding of consent – particularly around the use of secondary data and the difference between opt-in an opt-out."* Looking ahead it was proposed that *"new regulation will be influenced by others including the EU's GDPR highly granular approach[206] versus the US which is more hands-off."* The view was that the EU approach and its wider global influence could well prevail in most countries (beyond the US, India and China).

While some put faith in the ability of new privacy-enhancing technologies to address some of the core requirements, and so move ahead of regulation, by and large, the need for more proactive regulation around patient data is a common request and so one that should be central to many future strategies. In the US, *"to provide better services while dealing with the challenges of privacy and cross border differences in regulation and operating models"* is seen as no easy task.

CASE STUDY:

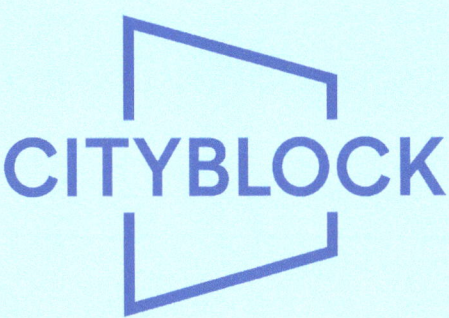

"We believe health happens locally, so we put individuals and their communities at the centre of what we do."

One of the most recent Alphabet spin-outs, Citiblock Health is focused on the poorest city dwellers – initially with a US remit. It is building a personalized health system concentrated on local communities and is seeking to more effectively provide health services to those on Medicaid or Medicare who have either fallen through the gaps in the system or are 'frequent travellers' to hospital which, on average, cost $10,000 per stay.

Aiming to send its own health-care professionals into people's homes and so avoid the need for early hospital admission, its core capability is the potential to mine data to identify and direct where care is most needed.[207] Linking together caregivers and clinicians with social services all within the day-to-day life of the city block, the core aim is to address medical, behavioural and socio-economic factors in an integrated manner and shift the care balance to prevention and community support.

Adopting shared-profit partnerships with payers and hospital systems, by redirecting spending towards prevention at the local, neighbourhood level, Cityblock's primary focus is on the 20% of Americans at the bottom of healthcare access and especially those that have complex and costly health needs.[208]

Launched in 2018 in Brooklyn, to support its model of developing personalized plans with which clinical teams can better engage with patients, it is building 'Commons' – a digital care management platform that collects structured data on medical, behavioural and social needs. Mixing a broad set of real-world data with the latest in predictive analytics technology, Cityblock Health is taking a bold approach to improving impact in one of the world's most complex health systems "improving the health of urban communities, one block at a time."

CASE STUDY:

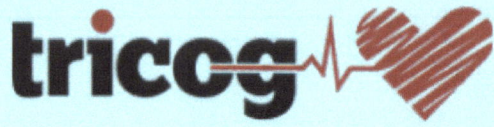

5 million Indians suffered a heart attack every year. India is one of many countries where it has been impossible to offer advanced heart treatment in poor villages, and, even if you could get an ECG, the local physician was not in a position to interpret it. Bengaluru based Tricog has fundamentally changed this and is now providing high quality analysis remotely. The company has built a cloud-based ECG machine and built a team of doctors providing 24/7 support from a centrally-located hub. Now any doctor at any remote location can take the ECG data of the patient and share it via the cloud to the Tricog team and receive expert advice within six minutes.[209]

Coronary heart disease is increasingly prevalent in India, having escalated from causing 26 percent of adult deaths in 2003 to 32 percent in 2013. In a nation where the doctor-to-patient ratio is one of the worst in the world with just 0.2 doctors per 1000 population (five times fewer that the US), delivering accurate diagnosis is therefore a major bonus. By adding a simple 3G communicator to a standard low-cost GE ECG machine, the company's platform collects physiological data and ECGs from medical devices in the field and then uses a specialized AI engine to process the data in real time and give the cardiologist an initial diagnosis. The cardiologist reviews the diagnosis and recommends next steps to the GP or nurse in the field instantaneously using the associated mobile app. A few specialists in Bengaluru can diagnose over 20,000 patients per day and provide the fastest and most-real time ECG analysis globally.[210]

Tricog was the first start-up selected for GE's Healthcare accelerator in 2016 and launched the same year. Coverage started locally in Karnataka and quickly expanded to Andhra Pradesh, Telangana, Tamil Nadu, Kerala, Maharashtra, and Delhi.[211] With product and the services offered on a pay-per-use model, so it also solves affordability issues for even small general practitioners, Tricog now provides access in 340 cities in 23 states, including in some of the most remote locations in India. It has changed the 80% chance that a heart attack will take a life to an 80% chance that the patient survives.[212] One of several Indian start-ups significantly improving access and highlighting how in partnership with human expertise, AI can become a 'force multiplier' in bringing preventative health care to everyone, rather than just the affluent few.[213]

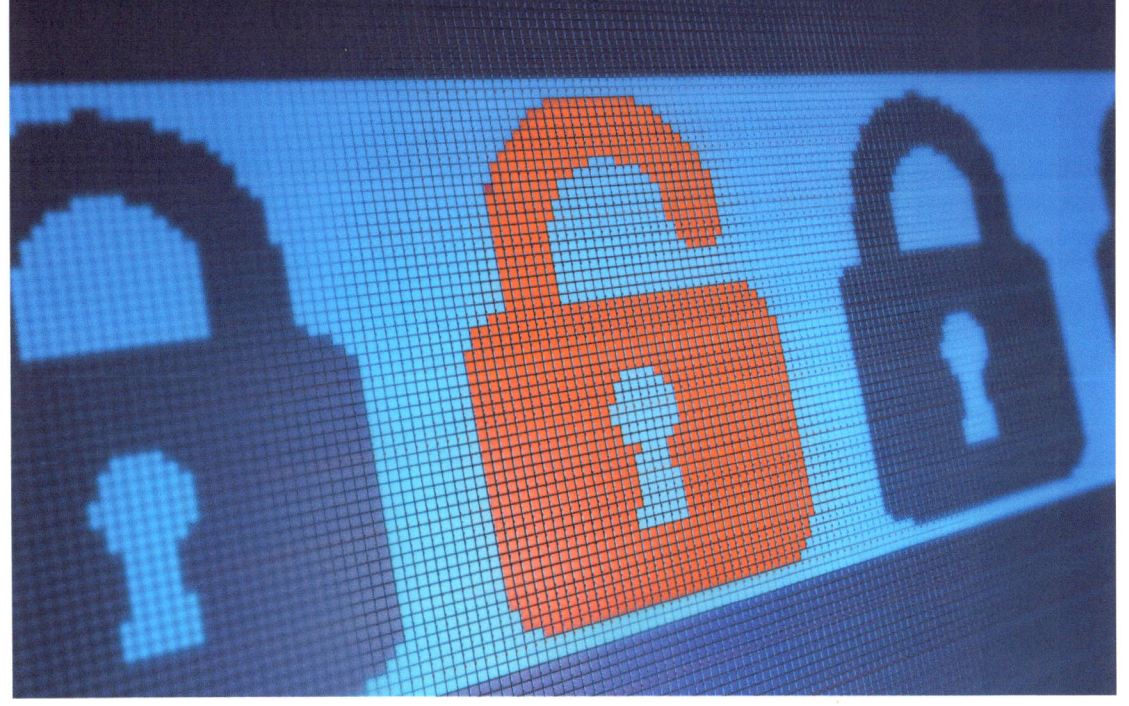

The privatisation of health information

The privatisation of medical knowledge and the increased use of new 'secret software' challenges the potential for healthcare data to be more open source or, at least, shared within an agreed governance system.

Many believe that more 'open' sharing of patient data has the potential to transform healthcare. But few seem to consider that it is a realistic possibility – there are just too many political and commercial interests at stake. Despite this, the ability to give a wide range of different organisations access to health information is an important element in many new models. Inevitably much could be available from a range of sources. Public healthcare providers often share data. It is also gathered by pharma companies from years of clinical observations and trials; some is controlled by the patient or an agent representative - social media and the app economy makes up most of the rest.

In general, however, there is little commercial appetite to share and most data is consequently stuck in some sort of silo. It hasn't helped that key regulations to set the standards for wider sharing have yet to be agreed. Despite the obvious benefits to society perhaps all this is unsurprising as, at a more mundane level, many established organisations are increasingly being threatened by newcomers from the world of technology. With deep pockets and huge ambition, they look set to challenge existing practises. In fact, they are already upping the ante by attracting significant numbers of experienced, data-savvy healthcare professionals - many of whom have cut their teeth in the public sector. Looking ahead, increased competition, certainly in the short term, looks likely to limit the amount of data sharing still further. Despite the hopes, some important health information may be increasingly protected and ring-fenced.

THE TALENT GRAB

Looking first at expertise, we see a growing anxiety about the wholesale acquisition of talent by technology companies. This was specifically highlighted as an issue in Singapore. Allegedly (according to Linked-In analysis) over 2000 leaders in healthcare research have moved over to big tech in the last year or so to work on the varied associated 'special projects'. Whether recruited by Amazon, Alphabet, Apple, Facebook, Microsoft or others, the concern expressed was that *"so much talent is being bought wholesale by big-tech that the implications for the wider healthcare systems are substantial. Hospitals and even pharmaceutical companies cannot compete."* Even if, in the unlikely scenario, big-tech's moves into healthcare do not deliver on their ambitions, the downside for healthcare generally could be significant. Parallels have been drawn to the *"wholesale recruitment by Uber of Carnegie-Mellon's autonomous vehicle expertise"* in 2014 and 2015. Carnegie had spent 30 years and many millions of public research dollars building world-leading expertise – think of Mars Curiosity Rover navigating its way around a planet on average 200m km away from ground control. *"Within one fell swoop Uber took the majority of this knowledge private and, even though paying super-high wages, in doing so arguably gained from decade of public research at a discount. The same may now be taking place in healthcare."*

In a 2016 Nature article[214] Eric Topol, author of 'The Patient will see You Now', voiced several concerns. Although recognising that *"migration of clinical scientists into technology corporations that are focused on gathering, analysing and storing information is long overdue,"* he and co-author, John Willbanks, also see a shortcoming. With large organisations like Google and smaller firms such as 23andMe owning the talent and also controlling the data as well as the methods to match this to the individual, there could be a *"fundamental shift in biomedical research and health care."* The problem, they argue, is that if undisclosed algorithmic decision-making, traditionally used by the tech companies, starts to incorporate health data, the ability of black-box calculations to accentuate pre-existing biases in society could greatly increase. There is a huge downside to this for *"if the citizens being profiled are not given their data and allowed to share the information with others, they will not know about incorrect or discriminatory health actions — much less be able to challenge them."* The recent shenanigans of companies like Cambridge Analytica have already shown the potential costs to individuals and society of the mis-management of data.

PRIVATE INFORMATION

Many we spoke to were also concerned about the harvesting of information – both indiscriminate and focused. Many have their hats in the ring. For example, Apple's ResearchKit allows anyone who want to use it to design data collecting apps and is consequently already gathering data from millions of people, while IBM Watson, and similar organisations, are sifting through petabytes of data and building up unique insights on the health of individuals. Moreover, 23andMe is now the holder of the world's largest repository of genomic data and companies like ancestry.com entice the pubic to buy an analysis of their DNA on the cheap but the company gets to own a record of it too – that it can then monetise. Others have highlighted more *"secret software"* that may be in development: interrogating health information in similar ways to others like Cambridge Analytica have been doing with personal data. Palantir Technologies[215] is just one of those now working on health data *"revolutionising how your organisation manages, analyses, and shares data, irrespective of scale, format, or federation."*

Meantime pharmaceutical firms have been acquiring and retaining clinical data for many years. Although many of them see that they are now 'losing' their lead as new tech gains the upper hand in more personal and contextual information. Topol and Willbanks believe that *"closer-data and closed-*

algorithm business models will hamper scientific progress by blocking the discovery of diverse ways to examine and interpret health data." Private capital and public good may be at odds: As of Dec 2017, Apple, Alphabet, Amazon and Microsoft alone had over $500bn of cash in the bank.[216] Their ability to privatise health is considerable. As highlighted in one discussion, in 2016, *"23andMe's fundraising of $115m was, for example, equivalent to more than 70% of the entire US federal investment in the Precision Medicine Initiative."*

In other discussions several healthcare providers, hospitals and insurers reinforced that they *"would not be willingly sharing patient data with competitors any time soon."* Even though big tech is seeking partnerships, many established payers and players are holding firm and seeking to protect unique information and insights. Indeed, some are becoming more protective and see building competitive advantage in keeping hold of healthcare information – further increasing privatisation in silos. Others see that this may be a red-line in the control of individual data. With GDPR in the EU and similar regulations elsewhere all coming into force, many see future friction between the public and private data and knowledge pools.

OPEN AI

In our Boston event there was a fervent debate about how this impacts the next generation of AI – especially in terms of what may or may not be open source. Some see that *"there are uncertainties such as the privatisation of medical knowledge as more investment in genomics and AI mean that it is no longer open source."* Within this, some assumptions are being made on the *"key characteristics of future AI in healthcare will be that it is ambient, global, open-source, patient-focused and include humans in the loop."* In the follow-on discussion, the challenges about whether or not AI knowledge will be open source and what the governance model for this should be was explored in more depth.

One standpoint was *"AI has to inherit policy from communities of interest such as patient groups - people you can trust, and so open source is key."* An alternative perspective considered if the AI data had been developed privately – *"why should it be made open? Several companies do not see how to shift AI to an open source model."* Within this some commented that *"the (US) Health Information Exchange model[217] is not working – maybe because it was constrained to just Google and Microsoft?"*

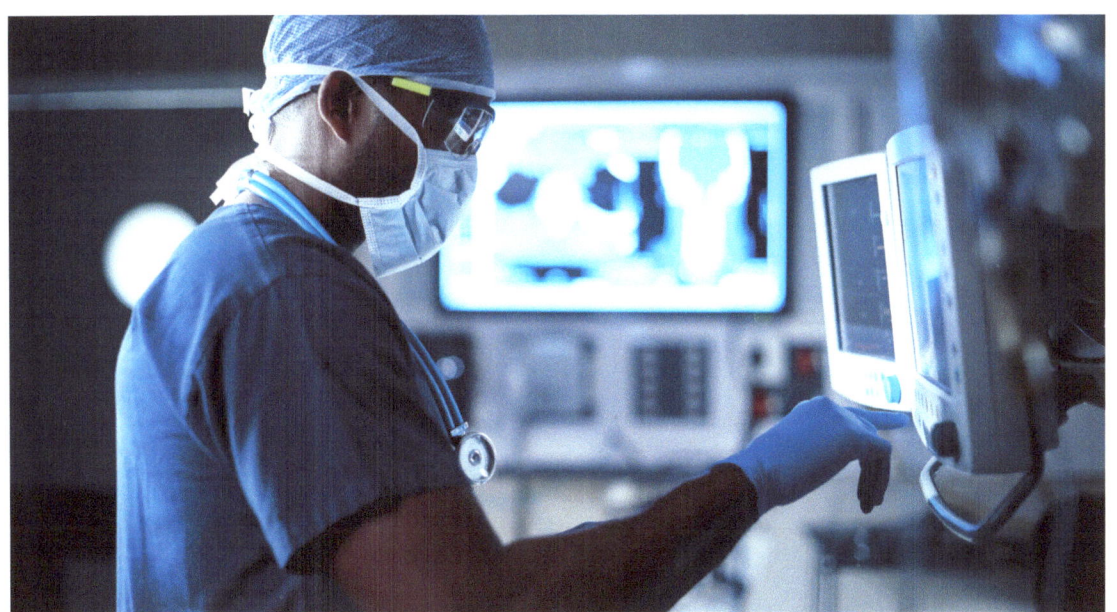

and asked whether or not *"HIPAA will continue to restrict data sharing between organisations and so limit the more open ideal here?"* Many recognize the need for greater collaboration and data sharing (or even data philanthropy) but point out that HIPAA is currently preventing this. One key difference highlighted in an AI discussion in Boston was the approaches that have taken by Apple vs. Amazon. *"Apple with its 'we will not see your data' (differential privacy) has had many benefits over Amazon which is listening and using your personal information. However, given there is a great incentive by AI teams to access and use more information, it may be that the Amazon approach wins out."* Apple's recent switch of policy on health data access may however change this.

There is clearly a divergence of views. Some companies who have made significant investments over the years in developing machine learning, cognitive computing and now deep learning believe that the hardware and software advances are their intellectual property and a source of competitive advantage - and so should not be openly shared. Others have either been open source from the start or have joined new open collaborations. Open source AI tools include Caffe at UC Berkley and Google's TensorFlow as well as Microsoft's CTNK and DMTK.[218] DeepMind regularly release open source environments, datasets and code to support and accelerate research in the wider AI community.[219]

One potentially significant collaboration here is the 'Partnership on AI' whose mission is 'to benefit people and society'. Founded by Apple, Amazon, DeepMind, Facebook, Google, IBM and Microsoft, part of its remit is to formulate best practices on AI technologies, to advance the public's understanding of AI, and to serve as an open platform for discussion and engagement about AI and its influences on people and society.[220] Widely praised as a welcome cross-sector collaboration at the early stage of a new industry's development, this may well emerge as a mechanism for more open sharing of health information. How far it will enable more data sharing is however challenged by some.

HOSPITAL DATA

One final notable view from Singapore was that, as global tech firms become more data-rich and influential in healthcare, *"hospitals will themselves want to develop / gain their own algorithms to use with their own data (that is not shared with others)."* This will then potentially enable them to be more accurate than the general AI systems developed by others. The high-quality, clinical data in hospitals will *"give them the advantage allowing them to provide better assessment (and prediction)."*

It appears as though the ownership and access to AI technology and specific algorithms may be influenced by just as many perspectives as the wider patient data arena.

As Topol noted[221] "during the 1990s, IBM abandoned its proprietary web server software in favour of selling services based around open source software." At around the same "open source Netscape prevented Microsoft gaining monopoly with Internet Explorer." Will we see a replay in the world of health data? Maybe? Maybe not?

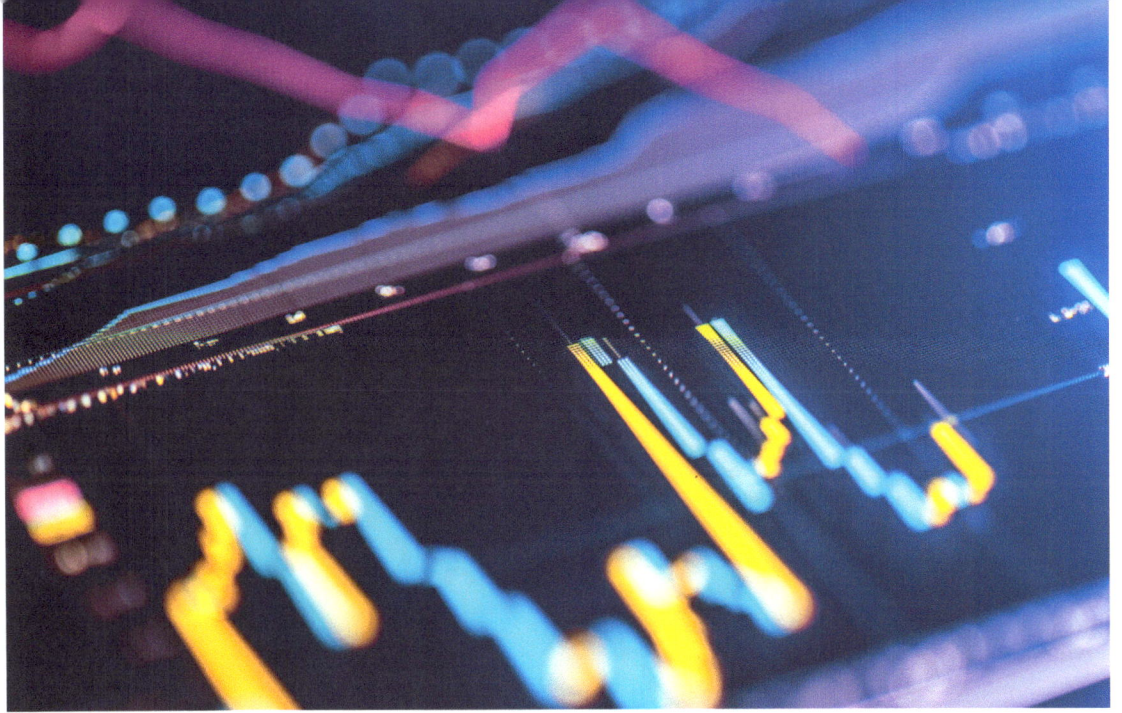

The value of health data

It is clear that patient data can be used to drive both social and economic benefit. As public understanding grows so will consensus about its worth. As this shift happens, those who can best grasp its multiple roles in, and value to, society, and render these things comprehensible to others, will likely have the more powerful voice.

Lastly, throughout our discussions, there has been an implicit view that patient data has value. As covered in the chapter on security and privacy, even at a mass level, hacked health data is worth more than financial data and can also be leveraged in more ways. The going price for a single record of financial information on a user that includes name, social security number, birth date, account information such as payment card number can range from $14 to $25 per record.[222]

With a reported street value of over $1000[223] the average US EHR is certainly a focus for hackers and, as we have seen, a legitimate, holistic, personalised health data set at an individual level is already worth more than that to interested parties. It is little surprise therefore that targeting US healthcare providers data is the top priority for many cyber-criminals. Equally, as addressed in the previous section, given this, there are many organisations increasingly seeking to privatise as much of it as possible.

More practically keeping patients in hospital is expensive and if data can be used to reduce these costs then many organisations are keen to explore its benefits. Some of the discussions in Boston focused on the potential changes that could be considered. *"It currently costs a hospital $2600 a day to provide a bed, and, in some cases, we are seeing hospitals pay care homes $500 a day to take*

117

patients out of hospitals. This is not the way the system is meant to work and shows why alternative reimbursement models must be explored." But is the discussion of value all about the money?

WHY THE CONCERN?

Within the current landscape, the advent of 'big' has changed our relationship with data. In particular, the meteoric rise of the so-called 'tech titans' whose business models rely on the collection, creation and monetisation of huge data sets, has thrust data to the forefront of social and political discourses around the world. These companies, whose products are now woven into the very fabric of our existence, have shown us what data can do and how it can transform our lives, but perhaps unwittingly, they have also pushed a topic once the preserve of 'nerds' and 'wonks' into the mainstream. Global public debates around everything from growing inequalities, to political freedoms and human rights, and the very future of economic and social progress, all now involve heady proclamations about the use, abuse, power and possibility of big data.

With the arrival of mass collection of 'personal' data, data *politics* is inevitable. It is the movement of data collection and analysis, experiment and discovery from remote processes, to the most intimate and fundamental parts of *everyone's* personal, social and economic lives, that has driven the idea of it into the heart of contemporary social and political conversation. Right now, debate about privacy is at the forefront of global discussion, but there are also those who are seeking to understand how new kinds of data might be used to address some of the biggest challenges in society.

No one doubts that patient data has economic value, the question is rather around how that value is exchanged and shared. But we should also consider the potential social value of health data, and how it might change the nature of the society's in which we live. *"Patient data has both commercial and competitive value – the principle of sharing this more freely is not going be an easy conversation to have."*

The optimists see that *"new platforms will seek to help individuals not only manage their personal information but also extract the best value from it – whether that be social, economic or health related."*

In Dubai, one negative future scenario saw that *"data mining and analysis will become expensive and data itself will become hard to access with less sharing than is really required for significant impact."* Moreover *"in this world, only data that has monetary value will be of interest and hence supported."* So, therefore *"we will focus on only the few, targeted conditions where impact can be made, or those for which the rich are willing to pay."*

If we are going to better manage the value of health data, then maybe we need a better shared understanding of what it actually is?

A CURRENCY?

To many of those we have talked to across multiple regions and topics *"data is a currency, it has a value and a price, and requires a marketplace."* But others are not so confident in this definition? Data can certainly serve as a medium for exchange, as it does when a consumer, for example, shares their personal data in exchange for so-called 'free' services. It can also be used as a store of value, even in quite a literal (albeit unstable) sense when it comes to crypto-currencies. So yes, data is like currency. But describing data as currency really doesn't tell us much. It just tells us that data has exchangeable value in certain contexts. In that sense, many things operate like currency. The economic value of health data might have risen in recent times, and more people might be aware of that value, but the same might also be said of quinoa. Describing data as currency simply edits out its myriad other features.

THE NEW OIL?

To others, there is another view that data is the new oil. As the Economist, for one, recently highlighted,[224] *"data is to this century what oil was to the last*

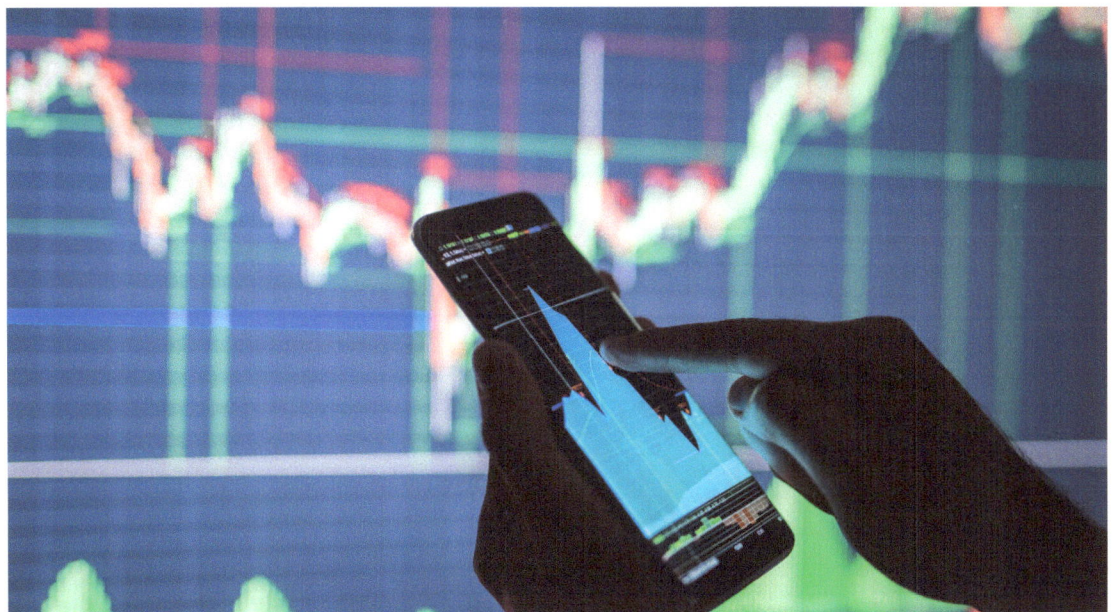

one: a driver of growth and change. Flows of data have created new infrastructure, new businesses, new monopiles, new politics and – crucially – new economics." Bloomberg and IDC have forecast the amount of data in the world to reach 45 Zettabytes by 2020 and 180 by 2025. The data majors of Apple, Amazon, Facebook, Google and Microsoft are now more valuable than the 20th century oil majors of Exxon, Shell, Chevron, Total and BP.

But again, is data like oil? Well, data is mined and refined, like oil. Vast hordes of it can make its owners (or 'controllers') very wealthy and powerful, like oil. We might even go to war over it, like oil. But there are also many ways in which data is not like oil. Data is not a finite, exhaustible resource, unlike oil. In many cases data is replicable or reproducible, unlike oil. The material costs of extraction, collection and movement of data are not high, unlike oil. The risks of data collection and use to society are real but not inherent to it, as they are with oil. In addition, as we have seen, data ownership is also not particularly easily defined, unlike oil.

These differences are important since they point to a completely different set of end-points for the data economy than there have been for the oil economy, and so demand a different set of societal responses. This metaphor blinds us, in fact, to the different options we have around how we, as a society, might *benefit* from data and avoid the calamitous potentials of its use, in ways that are simply not possible when it comes to oil.

The world's wealthiest companies are almost all now data-driven, or data-rich and the future of government looks set to be defined by 'smart' uses of large data sets. Great social value is also being created by the institutions of civil society, and a new breed of ethics-driven start-ups. Consumers and citizens are also now beginning to understand this landscape. Increasingly they are grasping the fact that what they once thought of as inconsequential personal data points, are actually being used to shape and define their lives at the very largest scales and are increasingly seeking ways to derive value for themselves from them.

As the volume multiplies and its quality improves, patient data is certainly going to become even more valuable in the next ten years. Healthcare organisations are already sitting on large stores of data that have significant value beyond the primary clinical use for which they were collected. Some are however reluctant to share what they have because they feel its value can be better used within their own ecosystems than by making it more widely available. They are also wary of exploitation by some of the larger, wealthier technology companies, hungry to enter the market. Others are, by contrast, still struggling to define what the value of their data really is, and are trying to understand which data-enabled outcomes to measure, and how to collect, analyse and share their findings.[225] McKinsey is not alone when it suggests that big data could transform the health-care sector, and many acknowledge that the industry must undergo fundamental changes before its full value can really be captured.[226] Lessons can of course be learned from any number of other data-driven revolutions where, all too often, players have taken advantage of data transparency by pursuing objectives that create value only for themselves and to the detriment of society as a whole. Given the global need for wider and more effective health care it would be a great loss to society if the industry did not learn from the mistakes of others.

Several of our experts felt that there is *"increasing honesty about the economics and value of healthcare and significant digital capability is being built within pharma."* But should we just be looking at health data's value through a financial lens? Isn't there *"a bigger picture view that should be driving our approach to the new world of more and better patient data?"* Moreover, are there not more enlightened ways to see value from data? Maybe more democratic perspectives? In Singapore, one view was that *"if the data value extraction can be democratised then this will open the door to information sharing at an extraordinary scale."* Our Toronto discussions highlighted the success of a system that *"has embraced evidence-based medicine where the focus is on the 'long run value' of healthcare."* Elsewhere the underlying sense that data has an inherent value (like oil) was challenged by the idea that *"health data itself is not interesting without context. More (like water) it can be valuable if it is in the right place at the right time."* Better patient data classification may be one solution providing insight between high value, low value and peripheral information.

Several organisations are now seeking to change the way we treat the value of patient data. For instance, Nebula Genomics' goal is to get the price of sequencing below $1,000 by working with biotech and pharma companies, which will subsidize a large share of the cost. In addition, users will be able to earn cryptocurrency in exchange for letting pharma companies use their data.[227] People who want to get their genomes sequenced through Nebula will pay with tokens, which will also be used by researchers and companies wanting to acquire that data. Initial modelling proposes that an individual could earn up to 50 times the cost of sequencing their genome – taking into account both what could be made from a lifetime of renting out their genetic data, and reductions in medical bills if the results throw up a potentially preventable disease.

THE SOLUTION?

It is clear that data can be used to drive both social and economic value. And, without getting lost in a metaphysical discussion about the concept of value, it seems safe to say that therefore the value of data lies in the uses to which it is put. Some of those uses seem to provide unequivocally *positive* value, such as searching for new cures for diseases. Similarly, there are some uses of data which seem to generate unequivocally *negative* value like identity theft, cyber-attack and data blackmail. Other uses seem to allow for the generation of both positive *and* negative value, at the same time.

Patient data, shared responsibly, can be used to help solve some of healthcare's most challenging problems. It can allow ideas to flourish and play a critical role in driving innovative research, deriving key insights and gaining new knowledge that can lead to faster and better treatments and cures for a wide range of health conditions and diseases.[228]

Similarly, whilst some argue that the principle of open data (particularly open government data) offers the best chance of unlocking the potential to solve societal challenges and bring collective benefit, others describe the exact same effort as giving away our most valuable assets to those with the best means to exploit it, whether or not they have the means to properly determine the best outcomes for society. The recent and controversial collaboration between the UK's National Health Service and Google's Deep Mind is a case in point. The partnership seemed to point towards exactly the kinds of optimistic hopes for big data sets and machine learning to help solve collective problems, whilst simultaneously sparking all of the worries around the potential harms of big data sets of personal information being collected and used by powerful stakeholders with inscrutable long-term interests[229].

THE FUTURE?

As many have stated *"data sets that contain information about human health are evidently hugely valuable."* At a time when health-care budgets around the world are stretched, payers are desperate for insights that might enable them to cut costs while maintaining quality.

Patient data and the uses to which it is put are set to define the future for societies and economies. We are going to see more data-driven companies, more data-driven social innovations, more cyber-security incidents, more breaches of privacy, more artificial intelligences, more miraculous transformations of the ways we live, and more dramatic consequences of that transformation.

In the short term, properly or improperly, many of the *mysteries* around data and its role in societal and economic change are going to disappear. Citizens, service users, consumers… people… *are* going to find a way to understand the value of their data (including their health data) to different organisations, and the different uses to which their data is put. This will happen regardless of debates about whether the way they understand it is technically correct or incorrect. This de-mystification is sometimes portrayed as a shift in power to the consumer, but it is really about a simple conveyance of understanding of big data from the few to the many, and it may happen regardless of where power or wealth ultimately comes to rest.

As this shift happens, those who can best grasp health data's multiple possibilities and realities, it's multiple roles in, and value to, society, and render these things comprehensible to others, will likely have the more powerful voice.

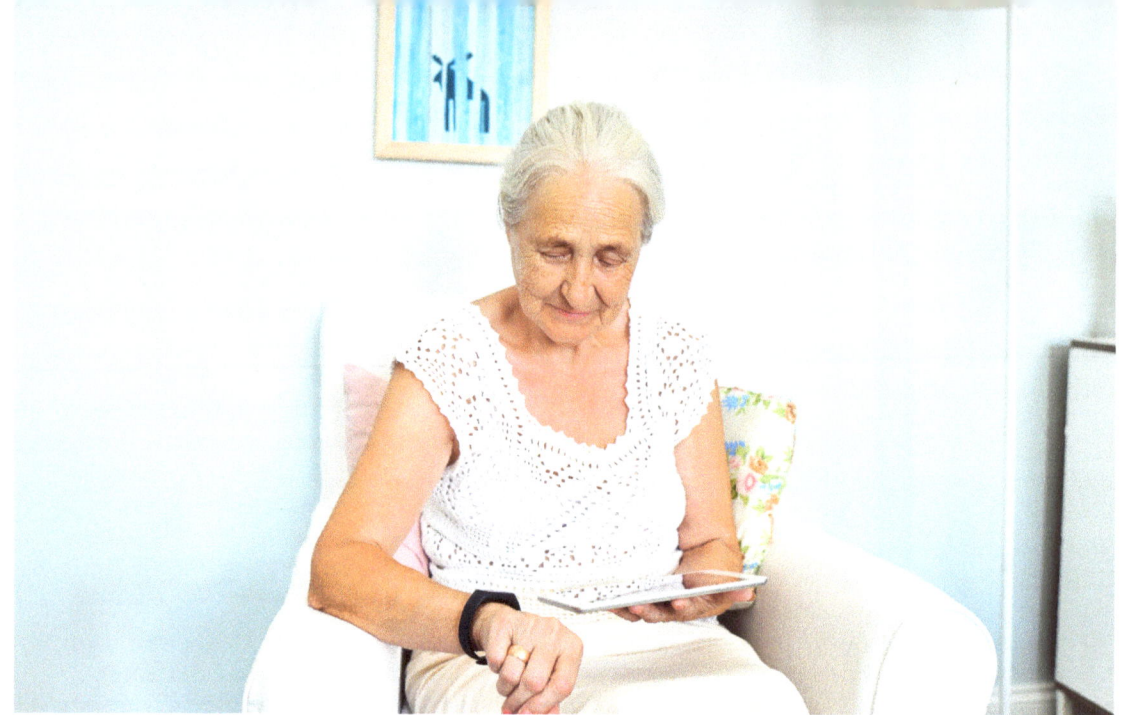

Conclusion

From all our discussions it is apparent that there is great potential for the future of patient data but also lots of challenges. There are many patient benefits as well as multiple additional opportunities for the broader community to bring to the sector. These may include hospitals, health systems and existing healthcare organisations, not to mention a host of new companies – many with deep pockets and sophisticated technology.

While there are many with global ambitions, for now it seems that change is most likely to occur at a more regional level. Whether because of data sovereignty, differences in privacy regulation or varied levels of trust in governments, healthcare providers and big-tech, it looks like progress will be in fits and starts with a localised or sub-sector focus. The end-goals of more widely shared information about patients driving a transformation in healthcare are credible and there is general agreement on the ideal destination, but the journey for many is going to be bumpy.

With all the developments in place, it is clear that healthcare is getting more personalised, more patient-centric and ever more data-driven. The investments being made across the sector by governments, pharmaceutical firms, IT companies and multiple new entrants not only support the direction of travel but are also building momentum. In some key regions there is both the opportunity for change and increasingly supportive regulatory environments that will encourage better integration, interrogation and control of patient data. China and India are, in many eyes, the ones to watch but equally other more mature and 'joined-up' systems in Europe, Australia, Canada and Singapore are showing promise. Questions have to be raised, however, about the US. The world's most well financed healthcare system is also its most fragmented and so, from a data perspective, the one with most silos. That said it is the home of many of the big-tech firms that are seeking to change the healthcare status quo and so, as they focus their resources and analytics on the tasks at hand, there are many that see tangible progress on the horizon.

While this report has highlighted a wide range of both opportunity and challenge, and has sometimes focused on the potential for the key players involved, we must not lose sight of the main motivation for most people in the sector – the better care of the patient. While some of the issues addressed here have covered the changing privacy and data landscape as well as improving efficiency and effectiveness and so reducing cost, few have relevance without delivering clear advantage for those who most need better healthcare – often the weakest and most vulnerable in our society.

If we can align the multiple strands of this issue, over the next decade, patients will:

- Become more involved in their overall health and how to improve it
- Be provided with more tailored support, diagnosis and treatment
- Have greater control of their health data, even if they don't own it
- Be active and not passive in the creation and sharing of value, and so
- Live longer, healthier and perhaps even happier lives.

If we get it right, these benefits will be delivered for the many and not just the few.

As a project, this has been a hugely insightful experience for us and judging from the feedback we have received, it has also been useful for many of those who kindly spared their time to join in the discussions. Once more we thank all those who participated for their time and enthusiasm.

This report is openly shared in partnership with multiple organisations around the world so we hope that its global context and multi-disciplinary perspective will help more to see the opportunity through an informed lens.

There may well be significant challenge but there is also huge opportunity. We look forward to seeing the potential change that so many have talked about successfully delivered.

To follow this project further and access more information please see www.futureofpatientdata.org

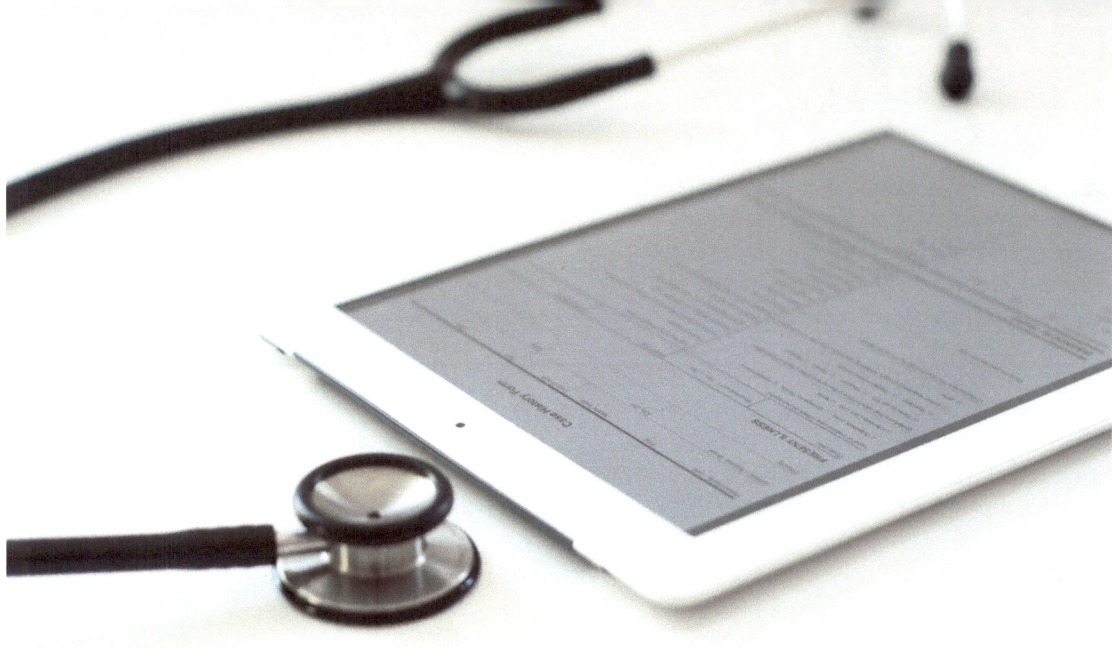

Questions

From the discussions and insights gained from this project, it is clear that the future of patient data is ripe with both opportunity and challenge. As we look ahead it is also evident that some organisations and governments are more ready for the emerging shifts than others. To help provoke further dialogue and discussion, we have suggested a number of questions that could be addressed. We use these, and other stimulus, as part of follow-on discussions with individual companies, healthcare systems and governments. They may also be useful to you internally to help further challenge assumptions and identify new areas for potential innovation.

Cutting across many of the topics covered in this report we propose 5 key questions each for governments, companies, hospitals and doctors as well as individual patients.

FIVE QUESTIONS FOR GOVERNMENTS

1. What are the greatest risks from sharing of public and individual citizen health data?
2. What regulation would help to control the use of personal data by others?
3. Where best can advances in data be used to drive down healthcare costs?
4. Which are the top opportunities to really improve public health?
5. Should citizens data be contained within national boundaries?

FIVE QUESTIONS FOR COMPANIES

1. How can you build and maintain trust in an increasingly transparent market?
2. Which of your datasets can create wider social value from being made open?
3. What is the best way to gain consent to share patient data?
4. Where can more information and better analysis most impact your business model?
5. How would a disruptive new entrant most effectively destroy your business?

FIVE QUESTIONS FOR HOSPITALS

1. How can you enable patients to understand how to best manage their health?
2. What patient data are you prepared to share with others?
3. How can you leverage personalisation and individual data to better treat individuals and also benefit the many?
4. What skill sets do you need to make best use of AI in the future?
5. How will new competitors capitalise from more private health data?

FIVE QUESTIONS FOR DOCTORS

1. In what ways will better data best empower your patients to take control of their health?
2. How will more accurate data help your patients better prevent illness or better manage their recovery?
3. How can you help your patients understand what their health data is telling them?
4. How can AI help to improve the care you provide to patients?
5. Where will be the most significant change in the doctor / patient relationship?

FIVE QUESTIONS FOR PATIENTS

1. Are you ready to take control of your own health data?
2. Do you think your data can really be private?
3. Who do you most trust with your personal information?
4. Which health insights would lead you to change your behaviours?
5. How much do you think your health data is worth and should you gain from it financially?

References

1. https://archive.opengazettes.org.za/archive/ZA/2017/government-gazette-ZA-vol-624-no-40955-dated-2017-06-30.pdf
2. https://www.chathamhouse.org/chatham-house-rule
3. https://www.cio.com/article/3174732/healthcare/unlocking-the-value-in-patient-generated-health-data.html
4. Boston event
5. https://www.wired.com/2014/11/on-sharing-your-medical-info/
6. https://www.stickk.com
7. https://www.agewellglobal.com
8. http://www.swordhealth.com/#/
9. London and Boston events
10. http://www.mobihealthnews.com/content/walgreens-shares-value-their-digital-incentive-based-activity-and-medication-adherence
11. https://community.fitbit.com/t5/Charge-HR/Daily-calorie-burn-goal-unattainable/td-p/1012542
12. https://www.willistowerswatson.com/en/press/2017/08/us-employers-expect-health-care-costs-to-rise-in-2018
13. https://www.bcg.com/industries/health-care-payers-providers/default.aspx
14. https://www.nytimes.com/interactive/2017/09/18/upshot/best-health-care-system-country-bracket.html
15. https://edition.cnn.com/2017/03/17/health/health-care-global-uk-national-health-system-eprise/index.html
16. https://www.theguardian.com/society/2016/feb/09/which-country-has-worlds-best-healthcare-system-this-is-the-nhs
17. http://www.commonwealthfund.org
18. https://www.theguardian.com/society/2017/jul/14/nhs-holds-on-to-top-spot-in-healthcare-survey
19. Mumbai event
20. Brussels, London and Boston events
21. https://techcrunch.com/2015/11/11/no-ui-is-the-new-ui/
22. https://www.brookings.edu/blog/techtank/2016/05/18/health-care-data-as-a-public-utility-how-do-we-get-there/
23. http://www.mckinsey.com/industries/healthcare-systems-and-services/our-insights/healthcares-digital-future
24. https://www.nap.edu/read/12212/chapter/6
25. http://www.himss.org/news/data-quality-strategies-improving-healthcare-data
26. San Francisco event
27. https://www.england.nhs.uk/2013/10/care-data/
28. http://www.wired.co.uk/article/care-data-nhs-england-closed
29. https://www.forbes.com/sites/theapothecary/2011/04/29/why-switzerland-has-the-worlds-best-health-care-system/#42deef907d74
30. https://www.ukdataservice.ac.uk/news-and-events/newsitem/?id=4615
31. http://www.mobihealthnews.com/content/depth-ai-healthcare-where-we-are-now-and-whats-next
32. https://www.nytimes.com/2018/01/24/technology/Apple-iPhone-medical-records.htm
33. http://fortune.com/2016/04/23/validic-healthcare-wearables/
34. https://validic.com/6-tips-to-thrive-in-the-conversation-economy/
35. https://validic.com/three-trends-for-wellness-leaders-to-watch/
36. https://www.philips.co.uk/a-w/about/news/archive/standard/news/press/2016/20160203-Philips-teams-up-with-Validic-to-integrate-personal-health-data-from-third-party-devices-and-apps-into-connected-health-services.html

37. http://pages.validic.com/rs/521-GHL-511/images/Validic%20HIMSS%20Analytics%20Research%20Paper.pdf
38. https://www.apple.com/healthcare/
39. https://www.cbinsights.com/research/apple-health-care-strategy-apps-expert-research/
40. http://fortune.com/2016/08/22/apple-acquires-gliimpse/
41. https://www.nytimes.com/2018/01/24/technology/Apple-iPhone-medical-records.htm
42. https://www.apple.com/newsroom/2018/01/apple-announces-effortless-solution-bringing-health-records-to-iPhone/
43. https://www.economist.com/news/business/21736193-worlds-biggest-tech-firms-see-opportunity-health-care-which-could-mean-empowered
44. https://arstechnica.com/gadgets/2017/11/fda-approves-first-medical-accessory-for-the-apple-watch-an-ekg-sensor/
45. https://www.economist.com/news/business/21736197-smartphones-are-increasingly-delivering-verified-treatments-diabetes-addictions-and-adhd
46. https://www.healthcaredive.com/news/apple-healthcare-future/511980/
47. http://medicaleconomics.modernmedicine.com/medical-economics/news/patient-records-struggle-ownership?page=0,1
48. http://www.health.wa.gov.au/circularsnew/pdfs/13318.pdf
49. https://www.finance.nsw.gov.au/ict/resources/nsw-government-data-and-information-custodianship-policy
50. http://www2.gnb.ca/content/dam/gnb/Departments/h-s/pdf/en/HealthActs/PrivacyQ%26A_Custodians.pdf
51. http://www.scot-ship-toolkit.org.uk/roles-and-responsibilities/your-responsibilities-data-custodian
52. https://www.sundhed.dk/borger/service/om-sundheddk/ehealth-in-denmark/background/
53. https://international.healthvault.com/gb/en/Howitworks
54. http://bmjopen.bmj.com/content/6/1/e010034
55. https://www.nhs.uk/NHSEngland/thenhs/records/healthrecords/Pages/what_to_do.aspx
56. https://www.nhp.gov.in/data-ownership-of-ehr_mtl
57. https://www.databoxproject.uk/about/
58. https://www.theguardian.com/science/2018/feb/18/genetics-how-do-you-make-money-from-your-dna
59. https://www.nebulagenomics.io
60. https://www.nebulagenomics.io/assets/documents/NEBULA_whitepaper_v4.52.pdf
61. https://www.technologyreview.com/s/610221/this-new-company-wants-to-sequence-your-genome-and-let-you-share-it-on-a-blockchain/
62. https://www.theguardian.com/science/2018/feb/18/genetics-how-do-you-make-money-from-your-dna
63. https://digi.me/mission
64. https://blog.digi.me/2017/05/31/digi-me-allowing-icelandic-citizens-to-download-their-own-health-data-in-world-first/
65. https://academic.oup.com/eurpub/article/16/1/4/527391
66. https://www.edelman.com/post/warning-signs-for-pharma
67. https://www.cognizant.com/whitepapers/healthcare-blockchains-curative-potential-for-healthcare-efficiency-and-quality-codex2995.pdf?
68. https://www.theguardian.com/science/2018/feb/18/genetics-how-do-you-make-money-from-your-dna
69. https://www.newscientist.com/article/2114748-google-translate-ai-invents-its-own-language-to-translate-with/
70. http://www.bbc.co.uk/news/technology-40483202
71. https://www.futureagenda.org/insight/human-touch

72 https://www.forbes.com/sites/davidshaywitz/2018/02/18/the-deeply-human-core-of-roches-2-1b-tech-acquisition-and-why-they-did-it/#e2d838e29c21
73 https://www.forbes.com/sites/davidshaywitz/2018/02/18/the-deeply-human-core-of-roches-2-1b-tech-acquisition-and-why-they-did-it/#e2d838e29c21
74 https://itunes.apple.com/us/podcast/tech-tonics-amy-abernethy-dosage-disney-data/id959413013?i=1000392676653&mt=2
75 https://flatiron.com/about-us/
76 https://www.forbes.com/sites/davidshaywitz/2018/02/18/the-deeply-human-core-of-roches-2-1b-tech-acquisition-and-why-they-did-it/#e2d838e29c21
77 https://itunes.apple.com/us/podcast/tech-tonics-amy-abernethy-dosage-disney-data/id959413013?i=1000392676653&mt=2
78 http://www.bbc.co.uk/news/technology-43033202
79 http://www.informationisbeautiful.net/visualizations/worlds-biggest-data-breaches-hacks/
80 https://www.csoonline.com/article/2130877/data-breach/the-biggest-data-breaches-of-the-21st-century.html
81 http://www.bbc.co.uk/news/technology-41753022
82 https://www.experian.com/assets/data-breach/white-papers/2017-experian-data-breach-industry-forecast.pdf
83 https://www.cisco.com/c/dam/global/en_uk/solutions/industries/healthcare-advisoryguide.pdf
84 http://www.bbc.co.uk/news/world-europe-41816857
85 https://www.mintpressnews.com/putin-questions-us-air-force-dna-collection-ethnic-russians/233946/
86 https://www.forbes.com/sites/mariyayao/2017/04/14/your-electronic-medical-records-can-be-worth-1000-to-hackers/#7f9edf3450cf
87 https://www.protenus.com
88 https://www.experian.com/assets/data-breach/white-papers/2017-experian-data-breach-industry-forecast.pdf
89 https://iapp.org/news/a/how-to-protect-patient-data/
90 http://www.bbc.co.uk/news/technology-40483202
91 http://www.eu-patient.eu/globalassets/policy/data-protection/data-protection-guide-for-patients-organisations.pdf
92 https://thewire.in/102349/without-data-security-and-privacy-laws-medical-records-in-india-are-highly-vulnerable/
93 https://www.dlapiperdataprotection.com
94 https://www.wired.com/2014/11/on-sharing-your-medical-info/
95 https://hbr.org/2017/06/11-things-the-health-care-sector-must-do-to-improve-cybersecurity
96 https://www.experian.com/assets/data-breach/white-papers/2017-experian-data-breach-industry-forecast.pdf
97 Boston event
98 https://www.england.nhs.uk/wp-content/uploads/2017/03/NEXT-STEPS-ON-THE-NHS-FIVE-YEAR-FORWARD-VIEW.pdf
99 Singapore event
100 https://www.healthaffairs.org/do/10.1377/hblog20170228.058958/full/
101 London event
102 https://atlantishealthcare.com/en-us/our-solutions
103 http://www.ukbiobank.ac.uk
104 https://www.23andme.com/en-gb
105 http://fortune.com/2017/02/21/craig-venter-human-longevity/

106 San Francisco event
107 http://www.toto.com/index.htm
108 http://fortune.com/2013/10/09/meet-japans-apple-of-toilet-tech/
109 https://www.mckinsey.com/business-functions/digital-mckinsey/our-insights/creating-a-successful-internet-of-things-data-marketplace
110 https://www.cio.com/article/3184575/business-intelligence/the-rise-of-the-data-marketplace.html
111 https://www.iqvia.com
112 Singapore event
113 https://coinjournal.net/new-partnership-seeks-create-blockchain-based-healthcare-data-marketplace/
114 https://hit.foundation
115 https://venturebeat.com/2017/11/28/iota-launches-iot-data-marketplace-envisions-devices-autonomously-buying-and-trading-information/
116 http://healthstandards.com/blog/2017/11/22/insilico-health-data-marketplace/
117 http://healthverity.com
118 https://medcitynews.com/2017/04/healthverity-raises-10m-for-dataset-marketplace/
119 https://www.coverus.io
120 https://www.huffingtonpost.com/entry/the-blockchain-based-health-data-marketplace_us_5a4f6a19e4b0cd114bdb3229
121 http://www.code-cancer.com
122 http://www.meaningfulconsent.org
123 London event
124 Brussels event
125 Brussels event
126 http://www-05.ibm.com/innovation/uk/watson/watson_in_healthcare.shtml
127 http://www.moorfields.nhs.uk/news/moorfields-announces-research-partnership
128 https://deepmind.com/applied/deepmind-health/working-nhs/health-research-tomorrow/moorfields-eye-hospital-nhs-foundation-trust/
129 https://deepmind.com/applied/deepmind-health/about-deepmind-health/what-people-are-saying-about-us/
130 https://www.babylonhealth.com
131 http://www.wired.co.uk/article/babylon-nhs-chatbot-app
132 http://allafrica.com/stories/201602161055.html
133 https://tricog.com
134 https://venturebeat.com/2017/11/26/ai-could-help-solve-the-worlds-healthcare-problems-at-scale/
135 https://www.asco.org/research-progress/reports-studies/clinical-cancer-advances/advance-year-immunotherapy-20
136 http://medicalfuturist.com/top-artificial-intelligence-companies-in-healthcare/
137 https://www.headspace.com
138 San Francisco event
139 London event
140 Dubai event
141 https://worldmedicalinnovation.org/wp-content/uploads/2018/02/Partners-FORUM-2018-BROCHURE-AI-Intro-180205_1332-HQ.pdf

142. Frankfurt event
143. https://www.economist.com/news/business/21725018-its-deep-pool-data-may-let-it-lead-artificial-intelligence-china-may-match-or-beat-america
144. http://studentlife.cs.dartmouth.edu/facelogging.pdf
145. https://arxiv.org/abs/1704.01074
146. https://www.techinasia.com/ai-chatbot-wysa-touchkin-penguin
147. https://www.fastcodesign.com/90128341/can-a-chatbot-be-a-good-therapist-this-scientist-founded-startup-says-yes
148. https://www.ft.com/content/6290297c-17c0-11e8-9376-4a6390addb44
149. https://deepmind.com/applied/deepmind-health/
150. https://deepmind.com/about/
151. http://www.zdnet.com/article/googles-grand-plan-for-health-from-fitness-apps-right-up-to-defeating-death/
152. https://www.theguardian.com/technology/2017/jul/03/google-deepmind-16m-patient-royal-free-deal-data-protection-act
153. https://techcrunch.com/2017/06/22/deepmind-health-inks-another-5-year-nhs-app-deal-in-face-of-ongoing-controversy/
154. https://www.bloomberg.com/news/articles/2017-11-28/alphabet-s-deepmind-is-trying-to-transform-health-care-but-should-an-ai-company-have-your-health-records
155. https://techcrunch.com/2017/06/22/deepmind-health-inks-another-5-year-nhs-app-deal-in-face-of-ongoing-controversy/
156. https://www.nanalyze.com/2017/11/8-startups-using-ai-for-personalized-health/
157. https://www.icarbonx.com/en/about.html
158. https://www.technologyreview.com/s/608987/how-ai-will-keep-you-healthy/
159. https://www.emarketer.com/Article/Health-Pharma-Marketers-Split-Digital-Spend-Between-Search-Display/1014123
160. https://www.cnbc.com/2017/09/07/facebook-held-a-breakfast-to-promote-clinical-trials-strategy.html
161. https://www.theguardian.com/technology/2017/dec/15/facebook-mental-health-psychology-social-media
162. https://www.economist.com/news/business/21736193-worlds-biggest-tech-firms-see-opportunity-health-care-which-could-mean-empowered
163. https://www.thememo.com/2017/08/09/signs-of-depression-instagram-social-media-mental-health/
164. https://epjdatascience.springeropen.com/articles/10.1140/epjds/s13688-017-0110-z?sf104446268=1
165. http://www.stgeorgeshouse.org/wp-content/uploads/2016/10/Digital-Health.pdf
166. https://www.economist.com/news/business/21736193-worlds-biggest-tech-firms-see-opportunity-health-care-which-could-mean-empowered
167. https://www.economist.com/news/business/21736193-worlds-biggest-tech-firms-see-opportunity-health-care-which-could-mean-empowered
168. Mumbai event
169. http://www.aravind.org/default/aboutuscontent/genesis
170. https:/www.wsj.com/articles/heart-surgeon-brings-high-tech-healthcare-to-the-worlds-poor-1442391424
171. https://uidai.gov.in
172. http://www.thehindu.com/news/cities/mumbai/news/linking-aadhaar-to-better-healthcare/article8288043.ece
173. https://indiamicrofinance.com/aadhar-healthcare.html
174. https://www.ft.com/content/5dfffdf2-f6f9-11e7-a4c9-bbdefa4f210b

175 http://ventures.mckesson.com/amazon-secret-health-tech-team-called-1492-working-medical-records-virtual-doc-visits/

176 http://money.cnn.com/2018/02/27/news/companies/amazon-health-care/index.html

177 Singapore, Dubai, London, Brussels, Toronto, Frankfurt, Boston and San Francisco events

178 https://www.ft.com/content/8929ecf4-0608-11e8-9650-9c0ad2d7c5b5

179 https://www.salesforce.com/products/einstein/overview/

180 https://verily.com

181 https://revenuesandprofits.com/how-google-life-sciences-verily-makes-money/

182 https://verily.com

183 http://fortune.com/2017/01/26/alphabet-other-bets/

184 https://revenuesandprofits.com/how-google-life-sciences-verily-makes-money/

185 http://www.zdnet.com/article/googles-grand-plan-for-health-from-fitness-apps-right-up-to-defeating-death/

186 https://www.cnbc.com/video/2018/01/09/verilys-project-baseline-google-maps-for-health.html

187 https://www.forbes.com/sites/chunkamui/2018/02/07/heres-how-amazon-could-disrupt-healthcare-part-2/#588730ee71e6

188 https://hbr.org/2018/02/what-could-amazons-approach-to-health-care-look-like

189 https://www.cnbc.com/2017/05/16/amazon-selling-drugs-pharmaceuticals.html

190 https://www.lab126.com

191 https://www.forbes.com/sites/shephyken/2017/06/17/sixty-four-percent-of-u-s-households-have-amazon-prime/#498ed5a84586

192 https://www.cnbc.com/2018/02/13/hospital-supplier-shares-dive-on-amazon-medical-supply-report.html

193 https://legalvision.com.au/what-is-data-sovereignty/

194 https://bfogp.org/blog/2016-04-all-your-internet-are-belong-to-us-on-nation-states-claims-of-sovereignty-over-ict-architecture-and-contents/

195 https://www2.deloitte.com/insights/us/en/focus/tech-trends/2018/data-sovereignty-management.html

196 http://indiastack.org/about/

197 http://www.bbc.co.uk/news/technology-42789282

198 Johannesburg, Oslo, Brussels and Singapore events

199 San Francisco event

200 http://www.pewresearch.org/fact-tank/2015/10/19/slightly-fewer-americans-are-reading-print-books-new-survey-finds/

201 https://www.pih.org

202 Sydney event

203 https://www.michalsons.com/blog/popi-regulations-popia-regulations/12417

204 http://indiastack.org/about/

205 https://www.oaic.gov.au/privacy-law/privacy-act/

206 http://www.keypointlaw.com.au/keynotes/impact-new-european-general-data-protection-regulation-australia

207 https://www.cityblock.com

208 https://www.cnbc.com/2018/01/04/alphabet-spin-off-cityblock-raises-20m-for-low-income-health-care.html

209 https://inc42.com/features/watchlist-healthtech-startups-2018/

210 https://venturebeat.com/2017/11/26/ai-could-help-solve-the-worlds-healthcare-problems-at-scale/
211 http://fortune.com/2017/05/03/tricog/
212 https://tricog.com/company-profile.html
213 https://venturebeat.com/2017/11/26/ai-could-help-solve-the-worlds-healthcare-problems-at-scale/
214 https://www.nature.com/news/stop-the-privatization-of-health-data-1.20268
215 https://www.palantir.com/wp-assets/media/capabilities-perspectives/Palantir-Health.pdf
216 http://uk.businessinsider.com/chart-us-companies-with-largest-cash-reserves-2017-8
217 https://www.healthit.gov/providers-professionals/health-information-exchange/what-hie
218 https://www.datamation.com/open-source/slideshows/15-top-open-source-artificial-intelligence-tools.html
219 https://deepmind.com/research/open-source/
220 https://www.partnershiponai.org
221 https://www.nature.com/news/stop-the-privatization-of-health-data-1.20268
222 https://securingtomorrow.mcafee.com/consumer/identity-protection/how-valuable-healthcare/
223 https://www.forbes.com/sites/mariyayao/2017/04/14/your-electronic-medical-records-can-be-worth-1000-to-hackers/#7f9edf3450cf
224 https://www.economist.com/news/briefing/21721634-how-it-shaping-up-data-giving-rise-new-economy
225 http://www.washingtonpost.com/sf/brand-connect/philips/wp/enterprise/how-data-can-inform-value-based-healthcare/
226 https://www.mckinsey.com/industries/healthcare-systems-and-services/our-insights/the-big-data-revolution-in-us-health-care
227 https://www.technologyreview.com/s/610221/this-new-company-wants-to-sequence-your-genome-and-let-you-share-it-on-a-blockchain/
228 https://www.healthitoutcomes.com/doc/the-monetization-of-health-data-0001
229 https://link.springer.com/article/10.1007%2Fs12553-017-0179-1

Future of Patient Data

Insights from Multiple Expert Discussions Around the World

www.ingramcontent.com/pod-product-compliance
Lightning Source LLC
Chambersburg PA
CBHW051911210526
45473CB00006B/1975